MIKE,
THANKS FOR
BEING MY BROTHER!

Refresh Life

oral health is the missing piece, adding years to your life, and improving your overall well-being!

Dr. Dan Sindelar

BALBOA.
PRESS
A DIVISION OF HAY HOUSE

Balboa Press books may be ordered through booksellers or by contacting:

Balboa Press
A Division of Hay House
1663 Liberty Drive
Bloomington, IN 47403
www.balboapress.com
1-(877) 407-4847

Because of the dynamic nature of the Internet, any web addresses or links contained in this book may have changed since publication and may no longer be valid. The views expressed in this work are solely those of the author and do not necessarily reflect the views of the publisher, and the publisher hereby disclaims any responsibility for them.

The author of this book does not dispense medical advice or prescribe the use of any technique as a form of treatment for physical, emotional, or medical problems without the advice of a physician, either directly or indirectly. The intent of the author is only to offer information of a general nature to help you in your quest for emotional and spiritual well-being. In the event you use any of the information in this book for yourself, which is your constitutional right, the author and the publisher assume no responsibility for your actions.

Any people depicted in stock imagery provided by Thinkstock are models, and such images are being used for illustrative purposes only.
Certain stock imagery © Thinkstock.

ISBN: 978-1-4525-3357-5 (sc)
ISBN: 978-1-4525-3359-9 (e)

Library of Congress Control Number: 2011904404

Printed in the United States of America

Balboa Press rev. date: 03/17/2011

Contents

Introduction

I would like you to join me on a very important journey. The message is simple: "your total health depends on good oral health!"

We will examine why this is so important, and then we will explore the new approaches that can completely change the way you "REFRESH YOUR LIFE." Oral health is the missing piece.

The research is mounting daily. Lack of ORAL HEALTH is a major risk factor to your body's total health. The mouth is where life begins. So when, where, how and why did the mouth become separated from the rest of the body? Medical research is finding oral bacteria to be associated with cardiovascular disease, stroke, cancer, diabetes, preterm birth, and Alzheimer's, just to name a few. What's reassuring is that we have ways to test for and prevent these potential killers...at the dentist's office.

The whole idea of Refresh Life is to open a door to your health, and then help you understand how crucial it is to care for your teeth and gums. I truly feel this is the new 'no smoking' cry for health. Bleeding gums may be as important to your overall health as not smoking, so you can see why we need to get this message out there!

Over the years as a dentist, I have noticed that most of my older patients in their 80s and 90s that were vibrant, living active lives, and had a lot of positives in their life, all had very healthy mouths. They had what I call young gums. I would often joke with them that they had the 'gums of a teenager'.

On the other hand, I noticed most of the older, non-compliant gum disease patients who took poor care of their oral health and refused any recommended treatment lived very unhealthy, disease-filled lives. They looked older than their age, and were almost never a part of the group of patients in their 80s and 90s. They always seemed to 'move on', passing away before they reached these decades of their life.

This is a pattern I've observed over the years, and with all the new revelations from research into deadly diseases being linked with oral health, you can see where I get my passion for this subject! Study after study confirms that good oral health is essential for our overall well-being, and lack of good oral health is proving to be a major risk factor to our health.

I hate to tell you this, but you probably have gum disease. In fact, the Guinness Book of World Records lists gum disease as the #1 most prevalent inflammatory disease in the world. Not only can gum disease kill you, 90% of it goes untreated. This has become a life and death issue!

Researchers have confirmed that gum disease is directly connected to the top two killers worldwide—heart disease and stroke. We are also seeing scientific clues pointing to other diseases being associated with gum disease, like diabetes, kidney disease, and Alzheimer's.

Are you surprised? The real question is why our advanced civilization would allow such a thing. Yet, periodontitis (gum disease) is more common than the common cold! Is it any coincidence that cardiovascular disease, diabetes, and stroke are also very common afflictions?

If we would take the surface area of the pockets around our teeth, the amazing thing is it would be the size of the inside of our forearm from our elbow to our hand. Try to imagine if it was bleeding and infected just like our gums often are. We would be rushed to the Emergency Room and treated Stat! And yet the same amount of area in the mouth is often overlooked. I'm here to say that with today's awareness of the Total Body Health Connection we can no longer ignore this!

You see, gum disease causes chronic inflammation. Inflammation is the body's first defense against infection, however when it is chronic, it can lead to a response in the body that brings on heart attacks, colon cancer, diabetes, stroke, Alzheimer's, kidney disease, and a host of other chronic and deadly diseases. I will look at this in greater depth later on, so you can understand just why something that is usually a good reaction for our bodies to have can turn so deadly.

Gum disease also allows harmful bacteria to enter the bloodstream. Gums infected with periodontal disease are toxic reservoirs of disease-causing bacteria. The toxins produced by the bacteria attack the gums, ligaments, and bone surrounding the teeth to produce infected pockets that are like large infected wounds in your mouth. The infected pockets give harmful bacteria access to your bloodstream, allowing it to travel throughout your body. These mouth bacteria are found to be responsible for many diseases and problems within the body, something that even a decade ago we did not realize.

The American Academy of Periodontology (AAP) asked the Center for Disease Control and Prevention to make monitoring oral health a priority as recently as August of 2010. Not only have studies shown that the rate of periodontal disease is 2-3x higher than formerly believed, the link between oral disease and general disease has been firmly established and must be made a national priority.

This is serious business. We need to wake up and see the connection of good oral health to our overall health. Gums are the early warning system that too few know to watch for!

The goal of this book is to bring about increased public awareness through education in order to diminish overall rates of disease in America...and around the world! My objective is to alert you to what's going on behind the scenes in your mouth in a way that will encourage you to make oral care a priority.

Let's look at a fictional account of an average American man. We'll call him Bob. Bob's father died after his third heart attack, despite everything the he could do—change of diet, regular exercise, keeping on top of medications and doctor visits. Bob's mother is doing well except for the awful rheumatoid arthritis that makes everyday activities a nightmare. Bob's wife has just been diagnosed with cancer and is preparing to undergo chemotherapy.

Bob's sons are both in their twenties, healthy and vital. The sad part is, they view what is happening with their parents and grandparents as just the way things are for aging human beings. I say it doesn't need to be this way. Of course these boys would pay anything for a cure, and they talk about making sure they stay fit and healthy, but they may be missing one key line of attack to avoid their own run-in with the same diseases that afflict the older generations of their family.

This book could help ease Bob's mother of her joint pain, and may have added years onto his father's life. It may also help Bob's wife survive cancer, and keep him from his own lengthy stay in the hospital. But most importantly, this book and its message could revolutionize the quality and *quantity* of life for those twenty-something boys. It could keep them from ever having to face an awful diagnosis of deadly disease.

See, there is one big message that I want you, dear reader, to get from this book. Whether you read on to learn more, or not; whether you care to take action on what I have to say...or not; I just want everyone to understand one simple thing:

Poor oral health will eventually lead to deadly disease.

Did you catch that? Let me say it again, real slow. **POOR ORAL HEALTH WILL EVENTUALLY LEAD TO DEADLY DISEASE.**

If you have gum disease, you are shortening your life and inviting deadly diseases to flourish in your body. This is now a proven and accepted fact, and my reason for writing this book is to bring awareness of how simple it is to prevent many of the health problems we see today. I want to offer solutions, simple solutions that anyone and everyone should do in their own bathrooms every day, and treatments they should ask for at the dentist.

Simply and clearly, good oral health is *essential* to your overall well-being.

My excitement is that if Bob's two boys maintain good oral health and guard against gum disease, they have a better chance of avoiding cancer, diabetes, brain abscesses, Alzheimer's, heart disease, stroke, arthritis, and more...simply by taking care of their mouths. Can you imagine the impact if their whole generation did this? Good oral health could lead the way to wiping out the diseases we have no cure for. Good oral health is the prevention!

What is amazing to me is that people still do not understand the sheer impact of this message. Today we have tougher laws on smoking and we protect workers and children from secondhand smoke. We place hand sanitizer everywhere to avoid passing viruses and germs. We walk and ride to raise money to find a cure for various maladies. Yet this message, despite now being fairly common knowledge, has no urgency to it. People still don't get it!

I have proof that this is so. Based on sales of dental floss, only 3% of Americans are flossing twice daily...3%! Yet this is the simplest way to prevent harmful bacteria from building up, weakening your gums, and finally entering your bloodstream. And these are the bacteria we find in the mouth of someone with gum disease and are associated with the very diseases listed above.

Poor oral health also affects the social aspects of your life, whether through bad breath or being ashamed of your smile. It could mean the difference between success and failure. The health of your mouth affects your entire life. It's that simple. If you keep your gums healthy, you help keep your whole life healthy.

Just over the last few years research has made huge discoveries in this area. It is now accepted that when your gums get infected with unhealthy bacteria, that bacteria affects your entire body and your overall health. It's not immediate. It takes time. So many of the diseases we associate with old age are because of a lifetime of poor oral habits.

I wish this was a book about curing heart disease, stroke, diabetes, cancer, Alzheimer's...to name a few...but it's not. This is a book about helping prevent those diseases from ever getting a foothold in your body in the first place. It's also about reducing the influence the lack of Oral health has on those same diseases.

I want to make a strong case for prevention through better and proper dental care, both at home and in the dentist's office. I want to wake people up to how important this really is. I want you to know what treatments to ask for in the dentist's chair, and why dentists often allow you to continue living with gum disease. I want you to be aware so you can make your own informed decisions.

Refresh Life is a concept, a path to a totally new 'wellness model' that reinforces the message of how everything is connected, and everything we do affects our whole body health. I believe that if we pay attention and take action, we can reduce these awful diseases that kill our loved ones every day! Change is possible. I want to show you how simple it can be.

Dentists are fond of the saying, "Only floss the teeth you want to keep." Which is funny, and truthful, but now we are seeing a much deeper and more serious side to this. Flossing isn't just going to save your teeth, it could save your life!

In this book I will teach you about Oral Systemic Health so that you can see the difference proper oral care will make in your life. I'm talking overall health as well as preventing killers like stroke, cancer, and heart disease. I will also speak about sleep apnea, and tell you my personal story of how oral care helped me. I will speak about food and diet, exercise, and spirituality, and how all of these things are connected to Oral Systemic Health. We will examine the problems, the consequences, and both current and upcoming solutions for better oral health.

There is a new awareness in our times of how interconnected everything really is. This book is about that, too.

Most importantly, however, even if you don't read a word past this introduction, I want to be sure you get my message: **good oral health is essential to your overall well-being.**

If that is the only thing you take away, and it encourages you to begin taking better care of your mouth, then I can be happy with that. But if you want to learn why, and what's being done to discover these connections, keep reading. If you want to understand how unhealthy gums could possibly be connected to having a stroke or heart attack, read on. If you want to learn about the research that's been done to find these connections, read on. Even if you are just on a quest to have better overall health, and teach it to your children too, please, read on. If there is anyone who can benefit to the fullest by proper oral care, it is the youth of today.

Chapter One

Why Refresh

Heart disease is the leading cause of death worldwide, yet many people with cardiovascular disease have none of the common risk factors such as smoking, obesity, and high cholesterol. So what is making people sick? You guessed it: gum disease.

Bleeding and inflammation anywhere will cause the liver to release C-Reactive Proteins. This is a natural reaction of the body that in the case of an injury makes good sense. However, a high level of C-Reactive proteins in your bloodstream is a strong predictor of cardiovascular issues...even more so than your cholesterol level! In fact, doctors today know that if you are being treated for high cholesterol, you should also be checked for gum disease and be seeking proper treatment if you have it.

Gum disease is one of the most common infections of humans, and these chronic infections are now shown to be directly linked to the "furring" of the arteries. The scientific term for this is atherosclerosis. Atherosclerosis is the main cause of heart attacks. Inside our arteries, the particular proteins produced from having chronic inflammation initiate atherosclerosis and help it progress.

These C-reactive proteins are also naturally produced after cells are exposed to other kinds of stress conditions that inflammation, such as exposure to toxins, starvation, and oxygen and water deprivation.

Because of this, the proteins are also referred to as stress proteins. They can work as chaperone molecules, stabilizing other proteins, helping to fold them and transport them across cell membranes. Some also bind to foreign antigens and present them to immune cells.

Because these proteins are produced by humans as well as bacteria, the immune system may not be able to differentiate between those from the body and those from invading pathogens. This can lead the immune system to launch an attack on its own proteins. When this happens, the white blood cells can build up in the tissues of the arteries, which causes atherosclerosis.

Researchers have found white blood cells called T cells in the lesions of arteries in patients affected by atherosclerosis. These T cells can bind to host stress proteins as well as to those from the same bacteria that cause gum disease. So the similarity between these kinds of proteins causes our body to turn on itself, and reveals the link between oral infection and clogged arteries.

This molecular mimicry means that when the immune system reacts to oral infection, it also attacks host proteins, causing problems for our arteries. Don't you think that information like this should fundamentally change our health policy? I feel it's time we stress the importance of adult oral health because of its connection or our overall health and wellbeing. Now that we see a direct link, controlling gum disease should be essential in reducing the risk of heart disease.

Words From Researchers

Professor Robin Seymour of Newcastle University Dental School, UK, is a leading oral specialist who finished an analysis of the link between poor **oral care** and coronary heart disease in May of 2010. His findings showed that unhealthy gums led to a higher risk of heart disease, with the key reason being that inflamed gums resulted in higher levels of C-Reactive protein. He also showed that dental cleaning had a profound effect, reducing the levels of C-Reactive protein in the blood and improving the health of blood vessels.

He also believed that most people are unaware of the strong connection between heart disease and gum disease.

"This is a significant step towards a more complete understanding of heart disease and improving treatment and preventive therapies," said Professor Seymour in an article written by medical journalist Susan Aldridge, PhD. "An understanding of all the possible risk factors could help lower the risk of developing heart disease and lead to a significant change in disease burden."

50% of all Americans have moderate to severe gum disease, and if what Professor Seymour says is true, most don't realize what an impact it can have on their health. So why aren't we paying more attention? This is a disease, not just an inconvenience, and we need to build awareness of how important good oral health really is.

Our mouth is the gateway to our bodies. We nourish, breathe, drink, and communicate with our mouth, yet somehow we all got sidetracked into thinking our mouth is not really connected to the rest of our body. We believe it is separate somehow, but research is fast proving this to be a mistake. America's door to better overall health is through the mouth first, precisely because everything is directly connected.

We cannot live without nutrients passing through our mouth. The moment we take a bite, our mouth starts processing our food through chewing and digestive enzymes. It's also a major pathway for our breathing, and the bacteria in our mouth (both the friendly and unfriendly kind) travel in the oxygen we breathe, the saliva-borne food and drink we swallow, and in our bloodstream.

Our mouth has a huge influence on our total health, and our overall lives. Despite this now being pretty common knowledge, most people are not taking action on it. Perhaps the message is not clear? Or maybe it is not urgent enough, not real enough to help us commit to

Science Daily (Jan. 9, 2008) Researchers at Howard University identified 11 studies that had previously examined clinically-diagnosed periodontal disease and cardiovascular disease. The team then analyzed the participants' level of systemic bacterial exposure, specifically looking for the presence of the bacteria associated with periodontal disease, as well as measuring various biological indicators of bacterial exposure. They found that individuals with periodontal disease whose biomarkers showed increased bacterial exposure were more likely to develop coronary heart disease or atherogenesis (plaque formation in the arteries).

better oral health care? What needs to happen in order for us to take it seriously?

Charles learned to take it seriously, and it changed his life... perhaps even saved it.

Charles had not been to a dentist in over ten years. He did not know he had any problems, and felt there was no reason to go if he was not in pain. However, he was struggling with his health. He was borderline diabetic, had blood pressure concerns, and high cholesterol.

He was found to have gum disease, bleeding gums, with pocketing. His oral DNA salivary diagnostics revealed he had numerous bacteria associated with gum disease, and several associated with heart disease.

Charles has a family history of heart disease, so he was very interested in reducing one of his major health risks in any way he could. He went through with treatment for his periodontitis, being treated by preconditioning with both a 1064 laser and ozone therapy, followed by scaling and root planing. Once these in-house treatments were done, he also used PerioProtect at home, something I will talk about later.

Here's the great news for those of you who do not like going to the dentist: all of these procedures are pain-free!

The outcome for Charles is an amazing story. He no longer has bleeding gums, his pockets have reduced to normal levels, he is no longer borderline diabetic, and his blood pressure and cholesterol concerns have improved. The man looks and feels much healthier! And the follow up Oral DNA testing showed a virtual elimination of the bacteria of concern.

There is nowhere else in the body that the outside and the inside of us collide so dramatically than the mouth. We are seeing more and more evidence of harmful bacteria gaining access to our bodies due to our poor maintenance of oral health. As we go through and look in detail at some of the things mentioned in Charles' story, you will learn why treating gum disease also has a positive effect on the body.

A Social Impact

It's neat to see that helping people with their oral health can also improve their social lives. There is a definite negative social impact if you practice poor oral health. Our smile is an extremely important part of our emotional and social health. People with better smiles tend to have better jobs, more social interactions, and generally more successful lives.

Our smiles are the most universally recognizable facial expression worldwide. A smile conveys happiness, confidence, an easy-going nature, a willingness to get along. A smile also reveals our teeth and gums. Researchers have found evidence that having gum disease will negatively affect your smile, sometimes even deterring you from displaying positive emotions because of embarrassment of how your smile looks.

Researchers conducted a test on subjects while they watched a comedy program. At predetermined measurement points, the researchers assessed three dimensions of each patient's smile: the horizontal width, the open width, and the number of teeth shown. They also noted when and how often a patient would cover their mouth. They even took into account each individual's perception of how quality of life is affected by oral health.

The findings proved that periodontal disease can impact a person's smile. The more symptoms of gum disease, like loose teeth and red swollen gums, the more likely the patient was to cover his or her mouth or limit how widely the mouth opened during the smile. And the more gum recession seen in the patient, the fewer teeth he or she showed when smiling. Even the way the test subjects perceived their quality of life as a result of their oral health was shown to directly correlate with the number of teeth they had that were affected by gum disease.

The study author, Dr. Marita R. Inglehart, explained how smiling actually plays a significant and essential role in a person's overall well-being. Smiling affects a person's social interactions because it affects their self-confidence. It also has an effect on how people perceive one another. Because periodontal disease is prevalent in such a large number of adults these days, Dr. Inglehart wanted to investigate the link between oral health and a person's smile. You can read about her study in Science Daily's April 1, 2008 issue.

Even the president of the AAP, Dr. Susan Karabin, is quoted as confirming the connection of periodontitis to overall systemic health.

"It is already widely known that periodontal disease is connected to systemic health," said Dr. Karabin. "These results help demonstrate that periodontal disease may affect more than just overall health. It can also impact actual quality of life, making caring for one's teeth and gums all the more important."

It seems the lecture many get at the dentist each check-up...floss your teeth!...is not an effective way to get this message out. Flossing and brushing are by far the first, easiest, and most affordable way to improve oral health and prevent tooth decay, gum disease. Yet statistics show that the large majority of Americans are not flossing. I hope that if I show just how important oral care is, and how it can prevent heart disease, stroke, diabetes, and more, that you will take action. You will floss, brush, rinse, and visit the dentist. You will tell your loved ones about what you've learned. The message will get heard.

"Researchers writing in the New England Journal of Medicine found that aggressive treatment of gum disease leads to improvements in blood vessel function which lowers the odds of having a heart attack."
How to Live a Longer and Healthier Life by David Hamilton, Best Life Oct. 2007

We need a new awareness. I compare this to how we once doubted the effects of things like smoking on whole body health. Heck, the ancient Maya believed smoking cured asthma! Now it's accepted knowledge that smoking is really bad for you. We need to get that same understanding and awareness that not flossing is just as bad as smoking!

With new awareness of how dramatically our oral health affects our overall health, I believe this is the health message for the new millennium. It might very well be the Golden Age of dentistry, as dentists become the front line of defense against disease, instigating a new standard of health care.

There is an exciting new movement in the dental world, a new mission of bringing awareness to the importance of good oral health. The American Academy for Oral Systemic Health is being created as I write this, with a mission of working to provide relevant evidence about oral disease and its connection to general health. The goal is to offer knowledge and information that will lead to improved health, healing, longevity, and wellness. These dentists, doctors, and other health practitioners are dedicated to working together for a healthier future. If you would like to learn more or join up, visit online at www.aaosh.com.

Refresh Your Life

I used the phrase Refresh Life for the title of this book because my intent is to provide a very positive book about refreshing your life.

Here's a question: what does the phrase 'refresh life' mean to you?

To me, fresh means it hasn't gone bad, it's still full of life and good for you. It's how we want our food. It's lack of decay, not dying, life sustaining. It is fresh water, fresh air, and fresh food. It's also feeling fresh, good, healthy, and full of vitality and energy.

Now let's look at the word 'life'. Life is what we want, what we need. It's why we are here, for without life we are not. Life is a force, it's our being, our soul, our spirituality. Life is our nourishment.

So then what do I mean by 'refresh'? It is making new, renewing, a new start. The prefix is the most important part of the message. Refresh is something that's better than before, and it's everything the way it's supposed to be. We 'refresh' our life by improving it and removing anything that impairs it. I believe we can all heal life, heighten life, and allow life to be fresh again simply by taking better care of our mouths.

All it takes is making a commitment for better overall oral care. What I recommend is not expecting perfection right out of the gate. Instead of trying to be absolutely right all of the time, be *mostly right most of the time*. If we floss most of the time, brush most of the time, eat right most of the time, exercise most of the time...well, it will all add up to better overall health.

Is it too much to ask? I hope not. And I hope I can convince you that what I am asking is truly in your best interest. It's not some plug for dentistry. It's not in the interest of spreading fear. It's a simple message backed by solid research and facts that can change the world.

Chapter Two

It's Costing You $$$

Okay, I'd like to cover some basic statistics and explanations. Firstly, what exactly is gum disease, and how does flossing prevent it?

Pay careful attention to this. If you don't floss every day, you're leaving 40% of your teeth surfaces dirty, coated with gummy bacteria that causes staining and yellowing between and around teeth. That overgrowth of plaque eventually leads to gingivitis, the first stage of gum disease, which creates inflammation, bleeding, and tenderness in gum tissue that can lead to gum recession and bone loss...which in turn leads to an older look because you see more spaces, and less and uneven gum tissue. This is where you get the quaint term for aging, 'long in the tooth. '

Matters only get worse from there. Gum disease can eventually cause the bones underneath to dissolve away. When gum disease begins to eat away at the bone, there are changes in facial appearance that cannot be fixed, even plastic surgery. In a recent study in the journal Plastic and Reconstructive Surgery, researchers found that bone loss in the jaw, as well as the eye sockets and cheeks, aged people in ways those cosmetic procedures that tighten and plump the skin can't fix.

So that's the effect of poor oral care on your mouth and face, in a nutshell. Now let's look a little further at the effects of poor oral health on the rest of your body.

> "Periodontitis, a bacterially-induced, localized, chronic inflammatory disease, destroys connective tissue and bone that support the teeth. Periodontitis is common, with mild to moderate forms affecting 30-50% of adults in the USA. There is now strong evidence that people with periodontitis are at increased risk of atherosclerotic CVD—the accumulation of lipid products within the arterial vascular wall." (Science Daily, July 20, 2009)

As we saw in the last chapter, studies now reveal a direct association between periodontitis and blood vessel dysfunction, heart attack, and stroke. Over the last few years this has been studied at great length, and from various standpoints. Enough time has passed in this research to show a more long-term effect. In one study it was found that participants who reported less frequent tooth brushing had an increased risk of heart disease compared with people who brushed their teeth twice a day.

What's important to understand is that gum disease is affecting us in two ways: through the body's natural reaction to the inflammation and the invasion of harmful bacteria originating in the mouth.

Our endothelial function is the thin layers of cells that line the interior surface of our blood vessels. Periodontitis affects our endothelial function in a negative way. The bacterial infection originating in our mouths invades the tissue around the teeth, causes tissue damage and bleeding, and thus enters the bloodstream. Periodontitis also triggers a low grade inflammatory response throughout the body that has a detrimental effect on the vascular wall (refer to chapter one for more information on this process). It also releases bacteria into our systems. What's been discovered is that the plaque in our mouths is the same plaque in our arteries. So we have the inflammatory response, and the bacteria, both creating a deadly response in our bodies over time.

As recently as 2009, scientists have also discovered a genetic relationship between periodontitis and coronary heart disease. Dr. Arne Schaefer of the Institute for Clinical Molecular Biology at the

Kiel University in Germany revealed a genetic variant situated on chromosome 9, which is shared between the two diseases. This means the genetic variation that is associated with the clinical pictures of both diseases is identical.

What I find relevant is that coronary heart disease is the leading cause of death worldwide, and periodontitis, which leads to the loss of connective tissue and the bone support of teeth, is the major cause of tooth loss in adults over forty years of age. They are obviously linked.

Dr. Schaefer's research shows a genetic basis for both diseases to illustrate how they are linked. Although there are people who still doubt the correlation between gum disease and heart disease, periodontitis must be taken very seriously, and diagnosed and treated aggressively as early as possible.

If you have gum disease, you need to take precautions regarding cardiovascular disease *before* you suffer a heart attack or stroke. That's how serious this is. As recently as 2009, researchers have begun recommending anyone with periodontitis to get evaluated for heart disease.

While scientists are still studying other links between periodontitis and atherosclerotic CVD, what is apparent is that inflammation in the gums is affecting the entire immune system. In fact, it has become accepted knowledge that inflammation of the gums is a noteworthy active contributor to many chronic diseases.

What is important to see is that the current evidence is strong enough that anyone with periodontitis should willingly be assessed for coronary disease. What I find frightening is that the cause of advanced gum disease is all too often inadequately treated early gum disease. As dentists, we cannot continue to misdiagnose and ignore the gum disease we see in our patients. If you have bleeding gums, then bacteria is infecting and entering your bloodstream. Several types of bacteria found in gum disease are incredibly pathologic, so in my office we have a motto: **zero tolerance for bleeding gums!**

Some Statistics

Remember the statistics I mentioned at the outset? 93% of people with gum disease are at risk for diabetes. Ninety-three percent. That's a huge number, and even more frightening because so many people do not even know they have gum disease. Everyone has a choice to make. Do you want to be the diabetic who eliminates their gum disease and lowers their health risk and their health care costs? Or one of those who dies because of untreated gum disease and uncontrolled diabetes? When it's put that way, it doesn't seem like so much trouble to floss, does it?

Remember, eliminating gum disease in people with diabetes lowers their health care costs by 15% per year. That's good news! Do you remember the bad news? If you have both diabetes and bleeding gums, your risk of dying increases by 400-700%.

Do you remember the statistic about arthritis? Gum disease is an inflammatory disease, and that chronic inflammation spreads to the rest of the body. Arthritis is an inflammatory disease of the joints. Do you see the connection? Who wants to be in pain all the time? Again, when you look at it that way, it doesn't seem like too much trouble to floss. Remember, over half of the people with rheumatoid arthritis have periodontitis.

Here's more:

- People with gum disease are *twice* as likely to die from heart disease and *three times* as likely to die from stroke.
- Bacterium from the mouth is found in brain abscesses.
- Gum disease and tooth loss increase the risk for Alzheimer's Disease.
- Pregnant women with gum disease have only a 1 in 7 chance of giving birth to a healthy child of normal size.
- Gum disease increases the risk for head and neck cancer.
- Harvard research states gum disease increases pancreatic cancer by 62%.

- People with gum disease have *four times* the heart plaque as those without gum disease.
- An estimated 8% of all cases of infective endocarditic are associated with periodontal or dental diseases.
- People with gum disease are *six times* more likely to suffer a stroke.

Am I scaring you yet?

Some Facts

Periodontal disease is a basic inflammation and infection of the gums and surrounding tissues in the mouth. An actual infection that leads to disease!

The bacterial plaque that is the main cause of the infection is a sticky, colorless film that forms on the teeth and then hardens into a rough porous substance. This is the tartar buildup that we have to visit the dentist to have removed.

If it is allowed to continue its life processes without disruptions, this substance releases toxins produced by the bacteria into the plaque, which eventually leads to a breakdown of the fibers that hold the gums tight to the teeth.

As the disease progresses, toxins and bacteria make their way down the tooth until the bone that keeps the tooth in place is broken down and the tooth eventually falls out.

Gum disease is an inflammatory disease, and medical research is finding the same bacteria in your mouth is involved in the following inflammatory diseases: cardiovascular disease, cancer, diabetes, Alzheimer's, cerebrovascular disease, stroke...the list goes on, and it's a long one. I know I've talked about this already,

> *Flossing is the new Viagra! Gum disease is also a circulation disease. The healthier your gums, the better your circulation, making for...yep, a better sex life.*

but it bears repeating. This is the biggest revolution in medicine since the Germ Theory of the 1800's. Porphyromonas Gingivalis, one of the bacteria in gum disease, is now being discovered in numerous systemic diseases like diseased heart walls and clogged arteries. That's proof positive...the disease starts in your mouth!

There are still those who are cautious of proclaiming this as absolute truth. However, the relationship between periodontal and cardiovascular diseases is strong. Porphyromonas Gingivalis is a confirmed significant predictor of myocardial infarction, the clinical term for heart attack. Our bodies are under attack both from harmful bacteria entering the body system from the mouth and from the chronic periodontal inflammation due to infection in the gums increasing the body's immune response.

Each year cardiovascular disease kills more Americans than cancer. What most people don't know is that while eating right, exercise, and quitting smoking are important, good oral health might be the most important step of all! The extended exposure to the harmful bacteria found in an unhealthy mouth will ultimately lead to cardiovascular disease.

Let's Talk Money

Maintaining a healthy mouth is also a wise financial investment. Obviously, if left untreated, gum disease will lead to even more serious and potentially expensive health complications. In fact, better oral care might even be a way to reduce financial stress for the whole country. Here's a huge example. In looking at the connection between low birth weight and premature births with mothers suffering from gum disease, one study found that proper dental treatment for over 1,600 pregnant women with periodontal disease could save nearly 14 million dollars in health care costs later. It might also save a lot of little lives, too!

The pattern continues. Another report showed that treating gum disease in patients with diabetes reduced their medical costs 10-12% per month. In 2007, a study in Japan looked at 4,285 patients over a 3.5 year time span. The patients were between the ages of 40-59. Researchers found that cumulative health care costs were a whopping 21% higher for diabetic patients with severe periodontal disease than those with no periodontal disease.

These examples give us a clear picture of how poor oral health is affecting the financial health of our health care system. Yet it is not something that is talked about.

I may repeat myself a few times in this book, but it is because I want to be sure the message is heard: prevention of periodontal disease is very important to overall health, social health, and even our financial health. Taking care of our mouths could prevent the diseases that are our number one killers. Furthermore, proper oral care in our health system will directly result in lower total health care costs.

Is all this not worth the effort of putting a little string between our teeth each night?

Chapter Three

It's Costing Your Health

I wanted this book to not only bring awareness, but also to educate and explain how this is all possible, and why we didn't really understand the importance of good oral health before. It is essential for change to actually take place that each individual understand why it is so important. This chapter will look at some basics regarding gum disease, and then look at the individual diseases that have been shown to be connected to gum disease one at a time.

First off, you need to be aware of how widespread the problem is. Approximately 75% of the adult population has some level of periodontal disease, according to the American Academy of Periodontology. Three quarters of our population! That's why I say to you, kind reader, that you probably have gum disease right now.

Worse news, however, is that during each and every stage of periodontal disease harmful bacterium from the infection is entering your body through saliva and blood. At the same time this bacterium invades our systems and causes its own problems, our body is also responding to the inflammation in the gums. This causes the liver to release high levels of C-Reactive protein in response. When the body is fighting the inflammation in the mouth, it causes other unwanted effects to the rest of the body, further acerbating the problem of the harmful bacteria also entering the system from the oral infection.

All of this combines to create a deadly cocktail of problems within the body, a laundry list of diseases we have fought and raised funds for and prayed for a cure for...and watched our loved ones die from. Meanwhile a large percentage of the population does not seem to understand the depth of the danger. We simply aren't aware of how much our poor oral care is affecting our health. The connection is clear, and the obvious solution is to care for the mouth in order to avoid these diseases.

The mouth is a reflection of a patient's overall health, harmful habits, and nutritional status. Our mouths reveal our addictions like smoking or having a sweet tooth. They show what sort of diet we consume. The oral cavity is a portal of entry as well as the site of disease for the microbial infections that affect our general health. I will keep saying it in every way I can think of in hopes that the message will truly sink in.

Laundry List of Disease

Of all of the diseases discussed below, oral bacteria and periodontal disease are now confirmed contributing factors, and I will illustrate the research behind that statement. In some cases, it may be the periodontal pathogenic bacteria or their associated cytokines that are the culprits. In other cases, it may be the secondary inflammatory response within the body that initiates or aggravates an underlying medical condition. Whatever the pathway, it is imperative that patients understand periodontal disease and how it may be treated or prevented in order to prevent or help treat the diseases listed below.

Stroke & Heart Disease

This definitely bears repeating: currently cardiovascular disease kills more Americans than cancer. Studies show that people with gum disease have a higher mortality rate and 23-46% increased risk for cardiovascular disease and stroke. If you are worried about being a statistic, then you need to consider the health of your gums.

In a review of 225 veteran outpatients, researchers found cardiovascular disease was more prevalent in patients with advanced periodontal disease than those with good oral health. In another study, the University of Buffalo School of Dental Medicine cites three specific types of bacteria commonly present in gum disease that were found to increase the risk of heart attack by 200-300%.

The connections between gum disease and heart disease are now so commonly known and accepted that cardiologists and periodontists are calling for joint treatment and education for both dental and heart patients about the correlation. Many dentists are now suggesting patients talk to their doctors about testing if they see advanced periodontitis.

Periodontitis is very destructive. It is quite literally an inflammatory disease of the supporting tissues of the teeth, and the specific microorganisms that cause periodontitis result in progressive destruction. Yes, you read that right: progressive, ongoing destruction that feeds on itself and grows worse if left untreated.

In coronary artery disease, a thickening of the walls of the coronary arteries happens due to the buildup of fatty proteins. Blood clots obstruct normal blood flow, restricting the amount of nutrients and oxygen required for the heart to function properly. This, of course, leads to a heart attack.

What scientists and medical researchers have discovered is that the harmful oral bacterium that comes from gum disease has been found to attach to fatty plaques in the coronary arteries and contribute to this clot formation.

When the oral pathogens and inflammatory mediators from periodontal wounds enter the bloodstream, they induce a chronic low-level bacteremia (the transient presence of bacteria in the blood). As we've looked at before, they also cause a systemic inflammatory reaction, releasing C-Reactive Protein

> *Oral disease and periodontitis has, for many years, been considered a disease confined to the oral cavity. It is only in the past several years that substantial scientific data have emerged that indicate that the localized infections characteristic of periodontitis can have a significant effect on the systemic health of both humans and animals. [From the Annals of Cardiac Anaesthesia, Ebersole JL, Cappelli D. Acute-phase reactants in infections and inflammatory diseases. Periodontol 2000;23:19-49.]*

and systemic antibodies. This inflammation triggers an immune response that causes inflammation or swelling of your arteries. This arterial swelling results in decreased blood flow through your arteries...the same arteries which are already stressed by the buildup of plaque!

Other studies have shown that gum disease leads to a higher white blood cell count, which is an indicator that the immune system is under increased stress.

But there is good news. Research published in the *New England Journal of Medicine* found that blood vessel function improved *significantly* in patients given intensive treatment for severe periodontitis, compared with those who had only the basic plaque removal and polishing and were sent home with the lecture to floss more often.

Improving your oral care at home will help fight these diseases, and having good oral health throughout your life effectively prevents them. If your gum disease has progressed further, then proper diagnosis and care at the dentist's office is crucial to avoiding clogging and inflammation of the arteries.

Proper care and treatment can reverse the nasty effects of gum disease on your body. That's the good news I want all of you to hear.

Cancer

Recently a multi-year study published in the Archives of Otolaryngology in May 2007 showed that for every millimeter of bone loss, the risk of tongue cancer increases more than five times. The study stated that chronic infections can possibly play a role in cancer, either as a result of the micro-organisms present or as a result of inflammation which can stimulate tumor formation. Again we hear the same message that we did when looking at heart disease.

We have already talked about bacteria entering the system through your blood and your saliva. But think for a minute about how saliva adheres to the water droplets within the air you inhale every time you breathe. These bacteria-laden water droplets now enter your lungs, causing pulmonary infection and pneumonia, possibly leading to cancers in the bronchial tubes and lungs.

Inflammatory mediators found in inflamed gums called 'cytokines' can also enter your saliva. As they too are aspirated into the lungs, they have pro-inflammatory effects on the lower airway, which can contribute to further pulmonary complications. This shows that even your lungs are affected by the health of your mouth.

Oral cancer, which is a catchall phrase that includes cancers of the mouth, sinuses, and throat, strikes over 34,000 Americans annually. More than 25% of those cases will die of the disease, claiming more lives than melanoma or cervical cancer.

But it may surprise you to find that it goes even beyond the mouth and lungs, which to me again proves the point that your oral health is connected to your body's overall health. The authors of a recent study in 'The Lancet Oncology' linked gum disease to higher chance of lung, kidney, pancreatic, and blood cancers. And did you know there is a 62% increased chance of developing pancreatic cancer, the deadliest of cancers, if you have gum disease?

No one wants the diagnosis of cancer. How exciting to discover that even this devastating disease could be prevented by taking better care of our oral health!

Diabetes

The following comes from a report detailing the story of a diabetic patient who made a commitment to better oral care. Before she underwent a series of dental procedures last year, Malcom's A1c level, which reflects blood sugar control, was far above the safe range. Now, since she has a new dedication to good oral care at home and is nearing the end of her dental treatment for gum disease, Malcom's sugars are closer to normal.

"I didn't make the connection that it could improve my diabetes," she is quoted as saying in the report. But recent research shows that uncorrected gum issues make blood sugar more difficult for diabetics to control. Diabetes, in turn, can cause or worsen gum disease.

In other words, if you have diabetes, you could get gum disease, and if you have gum disease, you could get diabetes. They seem to feed off each other! And sadly all too many of us haven't made the connection between our health and our gums.

The underlying mechanisms are not fully understood as of yet, but like I've said before, gum disease involves chronic inflammation--which can trigger insulin resistance, a hallmark of diabetes--and also bacterial infection. So when periodontitis creates wounds that allow the bacteria to gain access to the body, then the body reacts to the bacteria and the inflammation in a way that is a negative for blood sugar control.

"In diabetes...the body-mouth connection is clear cut. You would think that physicians would be telling their diabetic patients to make regular dental visits to head off gum disease and that dentists would be advising patients who develop persistent gum disease to be tested for diabetes."
The Washington Post, Sept. 3, 2008

Here's how it works for diabetics: ulcers and open sores in the gums become passageways for the proteins and bacteria themselves to enter the body's blood circulation. These inflammatory mediators, as well as some parts of the bacteria, prevent the body from effectively removing glucose, or sugar, from the blood. The higher level of blood sugar is known as poor diabetes control. Poor diabetes control leads to serious diabetes complications such as vision disorders, cardiovascular and kidney disease, and amputations, among other problems.

This shows clearly that maintaining a healthy mouth is crucial to treating diabetes and improving the overall health of diabetics.

So the real question is why doctors and dentists don't team up against diabetes? They are obviously fighting the same battle, and would have more chance of winning if they worked together.

Obesity

Obesity is the new pandemic, as far as many doctors are concerned. Americans especially have eaten their way to a new age of triple-X sizes and the conquest of the burger joint. So how does this relate to oral health, you might ask?

A recent study published as a supplement to the Journal of Periodontology found that obesity, independent of any factors such as age, race, gender, or ethnicity, is a significant predictor of periodontal disease. It seems that insulin resistance mediates the relationship between the two conditions (as we pointed out in the section above).

The data showed that the severity of tooth decay and loss increased proportionally as insulin resistance increased. The number of teeth lost also increased with greater insulin resistance. So again we see a problem that is both causing and compounded by poor oral health, just as we did with diabetes.

I have already spoken about cytokines (those hormone-like proteins that lead to systemic inflammation). Turns out those same cytokines also lead to insulin resistance. This illustrates how the links between obesity, diabetes, and poor oral health actually exacerbate the problems from each one.

Since this is such a pressing concern in our society today, later on I will look a closer look at obesity in the chapter about overall health.

Alzheimer's and Dementia

Chronic inflammation and the degenerative brain disorder known as Alzheimer's disease are now directly linked, which lead researchers to look at gum disease as a frequent source of that inflammation. Sure enough, losing teeth and gum disease at an early age is shown to increase the risk of Alzheimer's.

Studies have been done to examine lifestyle factors of more than 100 pairs of identical twins where one twin developed dementia and the other hadn't. Because identical twins are genetically indistinguishable, the study was able to seek out the risk factors that could be modified to help protect against dementia.

What they found was that the twin who had severe periodontal disease before age 35 had a fivefold increased risk of developing Alzheimer's disease. The findings showed that chronic inflammation can damage tissue, including brain tissue, which would contribute to the onset of a brain disorder.

The researchers stated that they considered periodontal disease as a signpost, not a cause, but should we worry about this distinction or simply take better care of our oral health? It's true that even the inflammatory link to Alzheimer's may involve several other factors, but the results of this study also show an appreciation that chronic inflammation in the brain was an essential part of the disease process.

Simply put, inflammation raises the risk of cognitive decline, and periodontal disease introduces inflammatory proteins into the blood.

Another recent study by the University of Kentucky searched for a connection between tooth loss and Alzheimer's and dementia. Using a Delayed Word Recall test, which assesses memory, researchers established that participants who did not lose teeth over the span of three years averaged significantly higher recall than those who experienced tooth lost during those years.

Clearly even our brains will function better if our gums are kept healthy.

Pre Term Birth and Stillbirth

Here's an example of where the health of a person's mouth could affect more than just that one individual. Researchers have found that having gum disease makes a pregnant woman several times more likely to deliver a preterm, low-birth-weight baby. The reason for this is that a labor-inducing chemical called prostaglandins is found in high levels in cases of severe gum disease. If you have severe periodontitis and you are pregnant, those prostaglandins could cause you to go into early labor, which of course is dangerous for the baby.

When you have gum disease, your body reacts to the infections in your gums by producing these prostaglandins, a natural fatty acid that's involved with inflammation control and smooth muscle contraction. During your pregnancy the level of prostaglandins gradually increases normally, peaking when you go into labor. So if extra prostaglandins are produced as a reaction to the bacterial infection in your gums, your body may interpret it as a signal to go into labor and your baby can be born too early or too small.

Insurance companies like Aetna and Cigna have begun covering extra cleanings for pregnant women. They also cover additional deep cleanings, known as scaling and root planing, for those with more severe gum disease. Early testing and tracking of the effects of these deep cleanings in such women showed reduced numbers of premature birth and low birth weight.

Studies have shown that bacteria commonly found in the mouth and associated with periodontal diseases are showing up in the amniotic fluid of some pregnant women. Amniotic fluid is the liquid that surrounds an unborn baby during pregnancy. Any disruptions in the amniotic fluid, such as a bacterial infection, may be dangerous to both the mother and baby.

As recently as May of 2010, medical studies have found new links between gum disease and stillbirth. The first documented case of oral bacteria actually causing a full-term human stillbirth occurred early in 2010 in California. Researchers were able to identify a bacterium called Fuscobacterium mucleatum in the mother's oral plaque samples. They also found this bacteria in the stillborn's lungs and stomach, but not in the mother's birth canal. This groundbreaking discovery suggests the bacterium was transmitted from the mother's mouth through the blood to the fetus, and the fetus died because of the bacterial infection and inflammation.

Bleeding gums are the entry point for over 500 different types of bacteria. This is how the bacterium enters your bloodstream, where they set up shop and do damage to your body. Is it any surprise that it would affect the baby growing inside?

It is so important for expectant mothers to take extra measures for good oral care. As I explained, live gum bacteria have been found in the placenta, where it can trigger a preterm response to give birth. There is an urban myth that it is normal for your gums to bleed during pregnancy. Remember that there is the bacteria in your plaque, not your fluctuating hormones, that cause gingivitis and bleeding gums. It is a sign of infection of the gum tissue, and it puts you and your baby at risk.

There are also several studies currently being done revealing the association between periodontitis and its effect on Endometriosis. Endometriosis causes problems with fertilization and reduces the likelihood of the patient conceiving. This brings to mind a story told to me recently of a young lady, in her late twenties. She and her husband had been trying to get pregnant for 5 years, with no success. Her dentist found that she had rampant gum disease. Once successfully treated for her gum disease, she proudly proclaimed that she was expecting twin boys!

Orthopedic Implant Failure

Orthopedic implant failure sometimes occurs due to an infection induced by oral bacteria. As I've explained repeatedly, (and will continue to do so to make sure the message is heard), when gums bleed, bacteria from the mouth enter the circulatory system. Once in the bloodstream, these bacteria can settle in and around an artificial joint, causing an infection around the implant that may result in implant failure.

Awareness of the risks associated with arthroplasty infection includes understanding that there is a potential risk of contracting an oral induced blood-borne infection around the artificial joint, and it is recognized by doctors in this field that good oral hygiene is essential. Further, while most dental procedures do not require a preventative antibiotic, this is a situation where it may be advisable. The oral healthcare professional and the orthopedic surgeon need to work together to determine the best course of treatment in a case like this.

Anyone considering an orthopedic implant, including a hip or knee replacement, should also book a periodontal risk evaluation and exam prior to surgery. In fact, many orthopedic surgeons now require a dental clearance before they will proceed with the operation. This way, any necessary treatment can be rendered well in advance of the orthopedic procedure, which lessens the chances of complications due to bacteria that originated in the mouth.

In osteoporosis and osteopenia, researchers are still not certain of a direct link with gum disease. However, both diseases are bone-resorptive. The bone loss in both periodontal disease and osteoporosis is magnified, either locally or systemically, by the activity of cytokines...those proteins and glycoproteins involved in cellular communication. In periodontal disease, bone loss around the teeth leads to loose teeth and subsequent tooth loss. In osteoporosis, the bone loss can affect the skeletal structure throughout the body, leading to fractures and other complications. It remains to be seen if there is a connection between the two diseases, despite their similarities, but it seems to make sense to take whatever precautions we can.

Kidney Disease

Because the bacteria associated with periodontal disease enters the body's circulatory system through the bleeding gums and travels to all parts of the body, it may cause secondary infections and contribute to the disease process in other tissues and organs. This has been observed in the kidney, for example.

Unfortunately, like periodontitis, chronic kidney disease is another health problem that is undiagnosed in a significant number of people, according to Dr. Monica A. Fisher of Case Western Reserve University in Ohio. Fisher and her associates used data from the Third National Health and Nutrition Examination Survey to identify 12,947 adults who had information on kidney function and at least one risk factor. The researchers found that subjects with periodontal disease and those with missing teeth were nearly twice as likely to have chronic kidney disease—60% and 85% respectively.

As more studies examine the connection between periodontal disease and chronic kidney disease, the information can be used to help decrease the incidence, progression, and complications of chronic kidney disease. Given the numerous shared risk factors for cardiovascular disease and chronic kidney disease, it makes sense that periodontitis is also associated with the renal insufficiency that causes kidney disease.

Too Many Signs

Whether the research confirms a direct connection or an additive effect, it seems to me that the proof laid out above is worth the effort to take better care of our mouths. Whatever the route oral bacteria may influence, it is in every patient's best interest to maintain their mouth in an optimum state of health.

Chapter Four

Refresh Your Sleep

In this chapter I would like to look at a couple of other less-directly related health topics. Why? Well, because the closer we look, the more we see they are still very much tied to the issue of oral care.

Sleep apnea and obesity are already linked, and of course must be considered in a quest for overall good health. Sleep apnea is another disease that goes undetected more often than not, just like gum disease and kidney disease. It is a dangerous disease that can be deadly. Thankfully there are amazing new ways to test for sleep apnea, and many new and innovative treatments available.

Sleep apnea became part of my life when I was diagnosed with OSA (Obstructive Sleep Apnea) many years ago. After a descriptive look at sleep apnea, I will tell you my story of discovery and treatment in hopes that it will help anyone reading that suffers from, or has a loved one that suffers from this breathing disorder.

Sleep Apnea

Sleep apnea, which can be life threatening, is the leading cause of disruptive snoring and excessive daytime sleepiness. It has also been found to be responsible for job impairment and motor vehicle crashes, high blood pressure and cardiovascular disease, memory problems and weight gain, even impotency and headaches.

In the previous chapter the first and largest section was about cardiovascular health. Sleep apnea victims lose up to twenty years of their life and are 23 times more likely to have a heart attack (as compared to smokers who are 11 times more likely to have a heart attack).

Research shows that when we reduce sleep from seven hours to five hours, we double our risk of cardiovascular death. So if we're going to look at overall health and preventing things like cardiovascular disease, then we need to look at sleep apnea. And if we're going to look at how common dentistry can help us to better overall health, then sleep apnea is one of those places where your dentist could be your new best friend.

Over time we have discovered that poor quality of sleep is just behind smoking in directly affecting our oral health. Through trials of my own with sleep apnea, I discovered a wealth of information that I feel I should share with you on this discovery of how to Refresh Life.

You see, sleep apnea is associated with heart disease, diabetes, erectile dysfunction, and stroke, just as gum disease is, so it very much affects our wellbeing and health. To make things worse from a dental perspective, 80% of sleep apnea victims are bruxers. Bruxism, from the Greek word for gnashing of teeth, is the disorder where people grind and/or clench their jaw during sleep. Bruxism leads to tooth loss. There are actually more people with sleep apnea than have diabetes, and only 1 in 10 sleep apnea victims even know they have it.

In fact, statistics say that sleep apnea will soon be the most common chronic disease in industrialized countries. Thankfully there are innovative technologies coming to bear on this problem that will not only treat sleep apnea, but will allow for easy and affordable home testing. This is really important, since most sleep apnea victims don't even know they suffer from the condition. In fact, this new outpatient diagnosis system was listed as one of the top 10 medical innovations for 2010. The device was described as "self-contained, reliable, at-home sleep-monitoring device for screening, diagnosing, and treatment assessment of sleep-related breathing disorders."

Approximately 10 years ago I was diagnosed with moderate OSA (obstructive sleep apnea). The process of finding out started with minor symptoms. I was tired most of the time. I would nod off at the movies or watching television. I knew I had a problem, but at that time, there were basically only two options available for treatment. I could undergo surgery or I could try the CPAP machine.

Together my doctor and I decided on a CPAP machine. I used it for several years with limited success. The machine was bulky, awkward, noisy, and inconvenient. It also left me feeling awful the next day. So I pursued several of the surgeries available, which unfortunately also resulted in little if any success in reducing my symptoms.

Then, approximately five years ago, they updated my sleep study, and they fit me with a new and improved CPAP machine. Unfortunately this also seemed to have limited success with me. Finally it was determined that when I bring my teeth together while I'm sleeping, my air passageway blocks, making it hard to breathe. I would wake up with the air from the CPAP going in my nasal passages and out of my mouth. So we tried fitting me with a head strap to keep my mouth closed. This also didn't have the desired effect on my sleep apnea.

Three years ago I decided to try out an oral appliance. Thankfully this dental solution was a great success! The oral appliance comfortably holds my lower jaw down and slightly forward, resulting in an open air passageway, allowing me to breathe freely while I sleep. I am no longer burdened by the cumbersome machine, nor do I face any more surgeries. The best part? I'm finally getting restful sleep, a big factor in overall health.

A Closer Look

There are three types of apnea: obstructive, central, and mixed. Seventeen percent of the adult population has OSA, or Obstructive Sleep Apnea. In fact, there are more sleep apnics than diabetics. OSA is the most common type of sleep apnea, caused by a partial or complete blockage of the upper airway which occurs during sleep. People with untreated OSA frequently stop breathing while sleeping, sometimes hundreds of times a night, and often for a minute or more.

96% of men and 65% of women with hypertension have OSA. Such prolonged high blood pressure becomes a major risk factor in cardiovascular disease. So you can see how important it is to look at the connecting afflictions that combined are a deadly cocktail: cardiovascular disease, hypertension, sleep apnea, and gum disease.

Central apnea occurs when the brain does not signal the muscles in the airway to breathe, and mixed apnea is a combination of both.

Sleep apnea also causes a lot of other problems for those who suffer from it. Sleep apnea victims are involved with many auto accidents and high divorce rates. OSA puts a lot of mental stress on the individual, leaving them depressed, sleep deprived, and mentally unstable. This leads to a lack of reasoning skills and accountability.

The most frightening thing about sleep apnea is you could have it and not be aware of it. Thankfully there are some signs to watch out for, like waking up choking and gasping for air, restlessness and frequent waking throughout the night, morning headaches, dryness or even soreness in the throat, and finally mood swings, forgetfulness, and a sense of just not being 'with it.'

Solutions include using a machine to help you breathe, surgery, and an oral dental device, such as with my own story.

CPAP is a machine that delivers air by means of a mask positioned on your face to keep an air hose on your nose while you sleep. CPAP stands for continuous positive airway pressure. It does take some time to get used to the device, and specialists have found that 50% of patients are non-compliant and don't use the machine regularly. Some estimates put overall long-term compliance rates as low as 30%. Specialists felt a better solution needed to be found.

Patients can be evaluated for surgical options, treating obstructive apnea with various procedures to reduce the blockage. However, many patients that have undergone surgery found minimal success in curing their apneic tendencies.

Oral appliance therapy involves having a dental device fitted for your mouth that is designed to keep the airway open and unobstructed. The appliance is as easy to wear as a retainer or mouth guard. There are many different appliances available, with over 40 of them approved by the FDA.

These oral devices reposition your mouth so the soft palate, uvula, and the back of the tongue do not block the airway once you relax into sleep. It also stabilizes the lower jaw and tongue, and increases the muscle tone of the tongue. One of my favorites is the Somnomed Appliance, which is FDA approved for mild to moderate OSA.

Getting Diagnosed

If you think you may have sleep apnea, it is important to talk to you doctor or dentist about it. Now that there are home sleep studies available to diagnose the problem, it is much easier and more affordable to be tested and properly diagnosed for this disorder. One of my favorite home testing systems is ARES by Watermark. It is easy, accurate, and less expensive than the alternatives. You wear the ARES on the forehead and sleep in your own bed. This is something even Dr. Oz has talked about on television!

Due to the fact that many people do not even know they suffer from sleep apnea, this is groundbreaking and newsworthy information, and worth checking into if you have any signs at all.

Obesity

Obesity is a medical condition where excess body fat has accumulated to the extent that it has an adverse effect on health. Being obese increases the likelihood of heart disease, type 2 diabetes, certain cancers, osteoarthritis, and breathing difficulties during sleep.

Obesity is a leading preventable cause of death worldwide. It is an epidemic in our country, and obesity is a dominant factor in 50% of all cases of Obstructive Sleep Apnea. If you are obese, you are probably a sleep apnea victim. To make matters worse, sleep disorders make it hard to lose weight.

In the last forty years, obesity rates in the US have doubled. The same studies show an increase in the average amount of calories consumed. Most of these extra calories are carbohydrates, and the primary source of these extra carbs is sweetened beverages. Pop, soda, whatever you want to call this poison, now accounts for almost 25% of the daily calorie intake for young adults. Instead of eating and drinking foods that nourish them, teens are consuming liquid sugar by the gallons.

Our fast-food mentality and highly preserved foods also contribute, and a sedentary lifestyle plays a significant role as well. In both children and adults there is a direct association between television viewing time and obesity. I'm sure none of you reading this are surprised by this data.

It has been discovered that the fat stored behind the abdominal wall is more harmful than the fat stored on hips and thighs. Some scientists believe belly fat secretes proteins and hormones that contribute to inflammation (that word again!), interferes with how the body processes insulin, and raises cholesterol levels. So again we see a health concern that is tied to inflammation, insulin, and cholesterol.

Excess weight around the middle combined with poor oral health greatly increases the chances of heart disease and stroke from the inflammation, and diabetes from the problems processing insulin and regulating blood sugar levels. Combine this with poor oral health, and we have a real problem that leads to high health care costs and devastating numbers dying from diseases that could have been prevented.

Live Healthy, Refresh Life

In a quest for understanding how to achieve better overall health, I felt it important to look at all the connections I saw happening, not just with gum disease, but with every systemic health problem that combined with gum disease could lead to such deadly results.

Chapter Five

Refresh Your Mouth

Okay, let's talk about basic oral care at home and in the dentist office. Unfortunately it is my belief that too many dentists are not recommending proper treatment for gum disease, or not treating it aggressively enough. Now that you are educated, you can ensure you get the care you really need to prevent disease in your body.

Some doctors today recommend that you request a C-Reactive protein test. High levels of C-reactive proteins are a warning sign of inflammation, and up till now they were considered a quiet killer. Now, we can be aware of these levels and understand the effect they have on our bodies.

> "C-Reactive Protein is the best crystal ball of health ever devised in a single blood test."
> Dr. Mark Laponis, Parade Magazine

Remember, proper treatment of periodontal disease reduces C-Reactive proteins levels by 25-30%, bringing a dangerous level to a more manageable level.

Possible chronic disease is not the only state that warrants extra attention to oral health. If you are going in for any kind of surgery, infection control is critical. These days a dentist's or periodontist's sign-off is often required before patients proceed to the operating room, especially for heart or orthopedic procedures.

Hormonal and developmental changes, too, can boost a person's risk of oral problems. Adolescents often have gingivitis due to a combination of raging hormones, orthodontics, and lax oral hygiene. Add any unhealthful habit--a study in the *Journal of the American Medical Association* found an increase in gum disease in young adults who were heavy users of marijuana--and the odds of oral health problems worsen still.

Facts about gum disease

Proper brushing and flossing is the easiest way to reduce and help prevent gum disease, but regular cleanings with your dental hygienist or dentist are also necessary to remove biofilm, plaque, and tartar build-up. Sophisticated techniques are required to treat advanced gum disease.

Gum disease can begin and progress without obvious symptoms, which is a situation similar to heart disease, diabetes, and cancer. Gum disease is an infection that can cause tooth loss and, as we've seen, is associated with several serious health conditions. An examination of your gums and jaw bones is the only accurate way to determine if you have gum disease. This includes measuring the depth of the gum pockets and using x-rays to determine the bone level.

The most common form of gum disease is gingivitis. It is distinguished from the more severe type, periodontitis or pyorrhea, by the depth of gum pockets and bone loss. If you have gingivitis, it is crucial to your health to get it under control before it can advance.

While genetics plays a role in gum disease, you can still have gum disease even though your parents and siblings were never affected by it.

Gum disease symptoms

Bleeding while brushing, flossing, or eating is a common symptom of gum disease. Not only does the bleeding indicate that the gums are inflamed, bleeding allows the bacteria in your mouth to enter your bloodstream.

While bleeding does not indicate how severe the gum disease is, or what level of treatment you will require, it is a red flag that demands your attention. Get the help of your dentist in deciding the steps that are necessary to reverse the disease, especially if it worsens.

The sad news is that the absence of bleeding when brushing, flossing, or eating does not mean you are in the clear. This is where an accurate assessment during a dental exam is crucial.

Even bleeding when the gum pockets are measured is indicative of gum disease but not its severity.

Gum recession, which results in teeth looking longer, is another symptom of gum disease. Loose teeth and shifting tooth positions where teeth no longer touch their neighbors are symptoms of severe gum disease. Tooth loss is a consequence of ignoring these symptoms. And please remember, these symptoms can occur with or without the bleeding that is so commonly associated with periodontitis.

The presence of any of these symptoms warrants a complete examination for gum disease by a dentist or periodontist.

What you can do about gum disease

Early detection of gum disease and treatment of gum disease can help you preserve your teeth, your smile, and your life.

Brushing and flossing every day is a very important behavior to prevent decay and gum disease. You should develop the habit of brushing and flossing every day. Your dentist and hygienist can help show you the proper way to brush and floss to ensure you are doing a thorough job at home.

Smoking is a risk factor for gum disease, oral cancer, and other diseases. No smoker likes to be lectured at, but you can prevent some pretty adverse consequences by quitting.

Bacteria are the prime etiological agents in periodontal diseases, and it is estimated that more than 500 different bacterial species are capable of colonizing in the adult mouth. Poor dental hygiene and periodontal infection have a major impact on overall health (yes, I said it again, and I will say it again still). The numbers and extent of harmful oral bacterium is directly proportional to the degree of oral inflammation or infection.

Plaque is a mesh of bacteria, biofilm, mucus, and debris coating your teeth. While brushing is effective in removing plaque from the outer and inner surfaces of the teeth, it is ineffective in properly cleaning the small spaces between the teeth. No big surprise, right? Still, amazingly enough, despite the facts we have on the importance of flossing, most people are not doing it.

That is why I had to write this book. I know that the more educated you are, the more you will understand how important it is to have good oral health. This way you will see the connections, and understand what is happening to your body when your gums get inflamed, and you will take action. That is my wish for you!

The purpose of flossing and brushing is to reduce the number of bacteria which inhabit your mouth. Normally, millions of these tiny bugs call your mouth home, feeding on food particles left on your teeth. These bacteria then produce acids as a result of their feasting and these acids contain sulfur compounds that can cause embarrassing bad breath.

Certain dentists routinely test blood pressure and refer patients to a physician if they find clues of systemic disease, and there's growing interest in expanding that aspect of dentistry. "We want to see the dentist become much more active in the role of diagnosis and screening," says Daniel Meyer, senior vice president of science and professional affairs for the American Dental Association.

Think of it this way. Brushing without flossing is like washing only 65% of your body...the other 35% remains dirty! If you do not floss and allow plaque to remain between teeth, deadly biofilm will thrive. Over time, dangerous types of bacteria build up within the biofilm and produce toxins which can cause inflammation and eat away at the gums and underlying supportive tooth structures, including the bone. This can lead to bone loss, loose teeth, and ultimately tooth loss...to say nothing of the bacteria that is entering your blood system during this process. Here in the United States, gum disease is the number one cause of tooth loss in adults.

New Awareness

Some dentists are forging ahead with new testing and treatments. Three years ago, Ron Schefdore, a dentist in Westmont, Ill., began testing adult patients' blood glucose, cholesterol, and C-Reactive protein (a marker of inflammation) before and after eight-week treatment regimens for periodontal disease. Monitoring those numbers helps him refer patients to a physician if something is out of the normal range. Another tool that inspires Schefdore's patients to commit to better oral care: a closed-circuit television. He zooms the camera in so "they can see all the blood and the yuck," he explains. "It really motivates them!"

I believe we will see a new level of communication between dentists and doctors now. Too many connections are being made every day between oral health problems and chronic disease.

We are so certain that dental procedures can introduce harmful bacteria into the bloodstream that antibiotics are often prescribed to susceptible patients before the procedures. One such problem is called endocarditis, which is an infection of the heart valve. Taking precautions like antibiotics is recommended for those with significant bleeding, or during periodontal surgery and scaling. It has even been shown that if unanticipated bleeding of a higher degree occurs, antimicrobial prophylaxis given within two hours following the procedure will be an effective prevention of such an infection.

Viridans streptococci bacteria are the most common cause of endocarditis following dental or oral procedures. Antibiotics such as amoxicillin, ampicillin, and penicillin V are equally effective, though amoxicillin is recommended because it is absorbed in the gastrointestinal track better and provides higher and more sustained serum levels. Those allergic to penicillins should be treated with alternatives like clindamycin hydrochloride.

Researchers have also discovered that one of the bacteria responsible for periodontitis, Porphyromonas gingivalis or P. gingivalis, actually works against your system. This bacterium knows how to enhance functions that help it and inhibit functions that hurt it. This discovery could impact how we treat periodontal disease.

How does this work? The P. gingivalis interrupts communication between complement protein C5 and Toll-like receptors (TLRs). These receptors usually notify a white blood cell of bacterial presence so they will destroy the bacteria. But P. gingivalis is really smart. It attacks the C5 molecule and changes it, activating the aspect C5a, which affects the communication between the C5 receptor and the TLRs. This impairs the ability of the cells to kill the bacteria. The P. gingivalis actually sabotages the immune system and promotes inflammation for its own survival.

In order to fight this communication breakdown, the C5a receptor must be blocked, inhibiting both inflammation and the persistence of P. gingivalis. If a way to effectively do this is found, it could translate into a way to prevent periodontitis and potentially other systemic bacteria disease.

Gum Disease – Take the Test:

While genetics plays a role, you can have gum disease even if other family members don't. After everything I've said here, it's pretty obvious how important it is to know whether you have it and what to do about it. Gum disease can be present without obvious symptoms, so having a professional examine you is the only definitive way, but in the meantime you can take the American Academy of Periodontology's 12-question risk assessment test to find out more about the disease and assess your chances.

You can also find this test online at: http://service.previser.com/aap/default.aspx where you can enter your answers and receive a report.

How old are you?

Your chances of developing periodontal disease increase considerably as you get older. Studies indicate that older people have the highest rates of periodontal disease and need to do more to maintain good oral health.

Are you female or male?

Studies suggest there are genetic differences between men and women that affect the risk of developing gum disease. While women tend to take better care of their oral health than men do, women's oral health is not markedly better than men's. This is because hormonal fluctuations throughout a woman's life can affect many tissues, including gum tissue.

Do your gums ever bleed?

There must be zero tolerance for bleeding gums. We refer to it as "ZT4BG", our little motto around the office. Think of gum tissue as the skin on your hand. If your hands bled every time you washed them, you would know something was wrong. However if you are a smoker, your gums may not bleed.

Are your teeth loose?

Periodontal disease is a serious inflammatory disease that is caused by a bacterial infection, and leads to destruction of the attachment fibers and supporting bone that hold your teeth in your mouth. When neglected, teeth can become loose and fall out.

Have your gums receded, or do your teeth look longer?

One of the warning signs of gum disease includes gums that are receding or pulling away from the teeth, causing the teeth to look longer than before.

Do you smoke or use tobacco products?

Studies have shown that tobacco use may be one of the most significant risk factors in the development and progression of periodontal disease. Smokers are much more likely than non-smokers to have calculus form on their teeth, have deeper pockets between the teeth and gums, and lose more of the bone and tissue that support the teeth.

Have you seen a dentist recently?

Daily brushing and flossing will help keep biofilm formation to a minimum, but it won't completely prevent it. A professional dental cleaning at least twice a year minimum is necessary to remove biofilm from places your toothbrush and floss may have missed.

How often do you floss?

Studies demonstrate that including flossing as part of your oral care routine can actually help reduce the amount of gum disease-causing bacteria found in the mouth, therefore contributing to healthy teeth and gums.

Do you currently have any of the following health conditions?

i.e. Heart disease, osteoporosis, osteopenia, high stress, or diabetes.

Ongoing research suggests that periodontal disease may be linked to these conditions. The bacteria associated with periodontal disease can travel into the blood stream and pose a threat to other parts of the body. Healthy gums lead to a healthier body.

Have you ever been told that you have gum problems, gum infection or gum inflammation?

Over the past decade, research has focused on the role chronic inflammation may play in various diseases, including periodontal, or gum, disease. Data suggests having a history of periodontal disease makes you six times more likely to have future periodontal problems. Periodontal disease is often silent, meaning symptoms may not appear until an advanced stage of the disease

Have you had any adult teeth extracted due to gum disease?

The more recent your loss of a tooth due to gum disease, the greater the risk of losing more teeth from the disease. Wisdom teeth, teeth pulled for orthodontic therapy or teeth pulled because of fracture or trauma may not contribute to increased risk for periodontal disease.

Have any of your family members had gum disease?

Research suggests that the bacteria that cause periodontal disease can pass through saliva. This means the common contact of saliva in families puts children and couples at risk for contracting the periodontal disease of another family member. Also, research proves that up to 30% of the population may be genetically susceptible to gum disease. Despite aggressive oral care habits, these people may be six times more likely to develop periodontal disease.

Chapter Six

Refresh Your Habits

Kind reader, now that I am done overwhelming you with facts and statistics, I hope I can offer some reassurance. I want to look at ways that oral health affects our lives beyond inflammatory disease. This book is about overall health, after all, and things like diet, exercise, spirituality, and meditation are as important as oral health in overall good health. What might be surprising to you is how connected all of these things are to oral health.

Before we get into solutions, I want to look at other less deadly ways oral health affects our lives

Bad Breath

A lot of people worry about their breath, and of course no one wants to be in close intimate contact with someone that has it. There are some surprising and not so surprising causes of bad breath.

The first obvious source of halitosis, or bad breath, is bacteria in the mouth. The stink-creating kind mostly hangs out on the tongue, happily churning out gases as they munch on food particles broken down by saliva. These bacteria multiply at night, when the salivary glands slow down, which is why bad breath is often present in the morning. H.pylori, the same bug that is often responsible for stomach ulcers, can cause bad breath and gum disease if it finds a permanent home in the mouth.

Medications like antidepressants, diuretics, and even aspirin can dry out the mouth, causing those bacteria we spoke about above to multiply. Even an excess of alcohol consumption will dry out your mouth.

Of course tooth and gum infections will cause bad breath, but so will respiratory tract infections like bronchitis, sinusitis, and even the common cold. Respiratory tract infections break down tissue, starting a flow of cells and mucus that feed bacteria that create foul odors. And potent breath can be a sign of more dangerous disease. Kidney failure produces a fishy smell, and uncontrolled diabetes creates a fruity smell on the breath.

Any condition that dries the tissues of the mouth, preventing saliva from washing away bacteria, encourages those bad breath bacteria to gain a foothold. Candidates for mouth breathing include sleep apnea victims, snorers, and asthma sufferers.

Diet, of course, affects your breath. Strong things like garlic and onion are well-known culprits, but foods that are high in protein or dairy products also cause bad breath because they generate large amounts of amino acids, which are perfect fodder for bacteria. A diet low in carbs burns stored fat, creating toxic-smelling ketones. Researchers have even linked bad breath with obesity, although at this time the connection is unclear.

Skipping breakfast is a good way to have bad breath. Eating first thing not only is good for body and mind, it stimulates saliva production and scrubs bacteria from the tongue...as long as it isn't a roasted garlic and onion sandwich!

Gently cleaning the tongue with a scraper is another method of keeping bad breath under control, since the area on the back of the tongue is the area most often responsible for bad breath. A tongue cleaner removes the bacterial biofilm, any debris, and the infected mucus. A toothbrush is not recommended for cleaning the back of your tongue because the bristles will only spread the bacteria around the mouth.

Chewing gum is a long-standing commercial way to improve your breath, and it does work better than mints (which only cover up the odor.) Sugarless gum increases saliva production, washing away oral bacteria that can cause bad breath. You can also chew on fennel seeds, cinnamon sticks, mastic gum, or fresh parsley, all common folk remedies. I recommend a green tea mint that not only refreshes your breath but is good for your gums and your health.

Of course I'm here to tell you that maintaining proper oral hygiene is vital to good breath. Would you be surprised to hear that flossing in particular will improve your breath? If there is rotting food trapped between your teeth that your brush cannot reach, then skipping the floss will only make that odor worse as the bacteria grows. Makes sense, right?

Looking Good No Matter Your Age

Are youthful looks important to you? Then consider that all the toxic waste from periodontitis ages the skin around your mouth much faster. It's not just a question of looking 'long in the tooth.' We are talking actual chemical changes to your skin.

Remember, flossing and brushing do more to fight the look of aging than plastic surgery. As gum disease progresses, you look older. First, you see more spaces between the teeth, and you see uneven gum tissue. Then, as the disease gets worse, the bone underneath can dissolve away, which changes your actual facial structure and makes you look older. Your cheeks and lips cave in, and wrinkles appear around the eye sockets, mouth, and cheeks. These are changes that cannot be repaired by plastic surgery, which can only tighten and plump the skin. And even if you opt for tooth replacement, there might not be enough bone left to place an implant in a way that will look appealing.

Missing teeth, even from the back where they are not visible when you smile, still affect your looks. Once a tooth is gone, the bones to either side immediately begin to shift. As the bone resorbs there is a loss of muscle attachment, which may result in the skin appearing saggy.

Some dentists even claim that dental implants are a better option than plastic surgery. By building up the jawbone and elongating the teeth, you remove wrinkles and create a youthful look while strengthening the bone within. This could eliminate the need for many facets of facial surgery.

Whatever lengths you are willing to go to keep looking young, it's important to realize that healthy gums and teeth will go a long way to preserving good looks and good health.

Chapter Seven

Refresh Your Soul

As we have discussed, our society is plagued with obesity. Being overweight often compounds the problems or even causes diseases like diabetes, stroke, and cardiovascular disease. Of course, this is a result of a diet of high fat, high sugar, low fiber, low vitamin D...a basic lack of the proper nutrients, which also affects the health of our mouth.

Not only will a diet of raw vegetables, fruit, proper fiber, and water intake improve our health, it will improve the health of our mouths as well!

Thankfully there are many lovely foods that actually promote better gum health. Studies show Kefir and yogurt are incredibly healthy for the digestive tract, and digestion starts in the mouth. We need to remember that digestion starts the moment we take a bite of food, not later on down in the system.

I believe starting and finishing each day with Kefir and yogurt really works to improve digestive health, and it's a program I utilize myself. It works! There are many more foods that help us in maintaining good oral health, and some of them might surprise you.

Green Tea

Green tea, among its other great benefits, has been shown to reduce gum disease. It also refreshes the breath. A recent study shows a component in green tea reduces the halitosis affect of porphyromonasgingivalis. I use Sencha green tea mints. Three of these mints are the same as one cup of tea, and are a great source of xylitol, which reduces tooth decay. The mints are vegan, sugar free, gluten free, and caffeine free. There are many other Sencha products such as tealeaves and snack bars that contain xylitol.

Sencha Naturals, the company which produces these products, wanted to explore other ways of utilizing this 'fragile yet potent plant called camellia sinensis.' Sencha is actually a particular grade of tea, and throughout Asia green tea is used in everything from toothpaste to gum to soap.

Not only is green tea loaded with antioxidants and polyphenols, research has show that green tea improves oral health because of the anti-bacterial and anti-viral agents that are known to kill oral bacteria. Green tea is also believed to boost metabolic rate without increasing blood pressure. For a simple cup of tea, that's pretty powerful stuff!

In 2009 a study was conducted in Japan that discovered men who drank a daily cup of green tea significantly lowered their risk of developing gum disease. The more tea they drank, the lower the risk. It is because of the antioxidants call catechins in green tea. These catechins hamper the body's inflammatory response to the bacteria that cause gum disease.

Dairy

You may be aware that including dairy in your diet can help maintain healthy bones and even promote weight loss. However, a recent study published in the Journal of Periodontology showed that those who regularly consumed dairy products such as milk, cheese, and yogurt also had a lower instance of gum disease.

"Research has suggested that periodontal disease may affect overall systemic health," said study author Dr. Yoshihiro Shimazaki of Kyushu University in Fukuoka, Japan. "This study reinforces what much of the public already knows—the importance of dairy in helping achieve a healthy lifestyle, including a healthy mouth."

Raisins

Here's the one that might surprise you, mostly because raisins are sweet and sticky, so most people would expect them to be bad for the teeth. However, research has shown that antioxidants in raisins fight the growth of a type of bacteria that can cause inflammation and gum disease.

Whole Grains

A study in the American Journal of Clinical Nutrition found that four or more servings of whole grains per day also reduced the risk of periodontal disease...by a whopping 23%! Refined carbohydrates like that found in white bread and white rice cause a spike in blood sugar. Whole grains such as oatmeal and brown rice are digested more slowly, causing a nice steady rise in blood glucose. Avoiding spikes in your blood sugar tempers the body's inflammatory proteins, and lowers the risk of both gum and heart disease, to say nothing of diabetes!

Antioxidants Are Important

Anything with a high level of antioxidants is going to be good for you and your gums. There are currently several studies on the positive effects of taking "Juice Plus" on Periodontal Health. There are many other things that are now being shown to improve oral health, like grape seed extract, which is one of many supplementary extracts taken for good overall health. The bottom line, however, is that the more raw food you eat, the healthier you are. Choose nuts, berries, raw fruits and vegetables, whole grains...you know the song and dance. Make small changes until they are a part of your everyday life, and soon you will see the benefits.

The Refresh Life System

When I set out to tell the world about this idea of refreshing your life, as a dentist it made sense to educate folks on the importance of oral systemic health. What became apparent very quickly in studying how everything fits together is that flossing and eating right were just the beginning. A non-active lifestyle goes hand-in-hand with obesity and poor overall care of our health...which includes oral care. So I'd like to also talk about the importance of exercise and stress reduction to the Refresh Life system.

As little as 10 minutes at a time can make such a difference, changing your whole outlook on life and self-care. The key to sticking to any exercise program is to make it fun. It has to be something you look forward to for it to become a part of your everyday lifestyle with ease. Include breathing techniques and some stretching, and now we are also combating stress!

Just like lack of activity and poor diet, both of which are common in today's society, stress adds to our overall poor health and lack of motivation to good self-care. We have cluttered our lives with stress. This brings about a lack of opportunity for peace and thoughtfulness, which we need for good health.

Stress hormones such as adrenaline and cortisol are exactly what our body needs in an emergency. Your heart pounds faster, muscles tighten, blood pressure rises, breath quickens, and your senses become sharper. This prepares you to face danger with increased strength and stamina, better reaction time, and better focus.

However, over prolonged periods of time stress stops being helpful and starts causing major damage to your health. Everything is affected, including your performance, your mood, and most especially your overall health. Chronic stress disrupts nearly every system in your body. Chronic stress can cause you to suffer from high blood pressure, a suppressed immune system, infertility, early aging, and an increased risk of heart attack and stroke. You may abuse alcohol or tobacco, both of which are bad for oral health. Long-term stress can even rewire the brain, leaving you more vulnerable to anxiety and depression, and less likely to take care of your teeth. You just stop caring. Worse yet, chronic stress is associated with higher and more prolonged levels of cortisol, and research shows that increased amount of cortisol in the bloodstream can lead to a more destructive form of periodontal disease. So again we see a health problem that both causes and is caused by gum disease.

And again we are looking at problems that plague our society as a whole, and we see that these diseases are the result of many different factors that all contribute: poor diet, high stress, lack of activity, and poor oral health. Our stressful lives again increase our likelihood for disease. I would say our current practices are no longer acceptable!

Better Gum Line, Better Bottom Line

Reducing stress in an effort to avoid gum disease may not only help sustain your overall health, but it might help your pocketbook as well. In a 2007 study published in the Journal of Periodontology, researchers found that preventing periodontal disease may be the one way to help lower your total health care expenses. After all I've told you, I'm sure you're not surprised! But here are some statistics to back it up: health care costs for patients with severe periodontal disease were 21% higher than those without periodontal disease. Because preventing gum disease may help reduce overall health care expenses, to say nothing of reducing illness, maintaining a healthy mouth may actually be a stress reliever in itself.

If you lead a high stress life, as most of us do, consider trying meditation CDs, or learning proper breathing techniques that you can practice each day. Remember, oxygen is life, and things that do not like oxygen are usually bad for us. We must bring oxygen into our bodies and ensure it is circulating to the brain in order to be able to function in a crazy world.

Here's a book I highly recommend. It's called "The Joy of Living" by Yongey Mingyur Rinpoche, who is a Tibetan Buddhist monk.

Mostly Right Most of the Time

All of this might start to be overwhelming. Please don't try to be absolutely right all the time (which will end up being none of the time), but instead be mostly right most of the time. Go for a walk on your lunch break. Eat a raw veggie plate for lunch instead of a sandwich or burger. Gently increase the serving of vegetables on your plate at dinner. Take time to care for yourself, whether that be a better night's sleep, listening to some great music, or booking a visit to the dentist. And take the time to floss each day.

The only way we will find total body health is to recognize how all of these separate things are actually connected and affect our well being as a whole.

Chapter Eight

Biofilm Is The Enemy

Biofilm is something you should understand if we are going to talk about gum disease and bacteria and systemic health. The studies of biofilms and how they work is also showing us why some diseases are so resistant to treatment, and what we might be able to do about it. We will also look at where biofilms are found and why you should care.

Biofilm is also a big concern for dentists and their offices. New advances are being made in both treatment options and awareness of how biofilms could affect the tools the dentist office is using to clean our teeth.

What Is Biofilm?

Biofilm is mass of microorganisms where the cells adhere to each other, and often to a surface as well. Most bacteria in nature exist in communities of biofilms. These structures serve as physical barriers and can severely limit the effect of antibacterial agents.

Scientists once studied bacteria by looking at cells suspended in a water droplet. Now they understand that disease-causing bacteria do not exist as isolated cells, such as in that water droplet, but instead create organized colonies or communities. These diverse communities are the biofilms. The most recent research shows that bacteria prefer living in these communities, and that the microbial biofilms are naturally tolerant of antibiotic doses 1,000 times greater than the dose that would kill planktonic bacteria.

You can learn more about biofilm at the Center for Biofilm Engineering, http://www.biofilm.montana.edu/

This is truly important research. It has been discovered that oral biofilm, once let loose in the bloodstream, makes a protein known as PadA which forces platelets in the blood to stick together and clot. This encases the bacteria, providing a further protective cover not only from the immune system, but also from antibiotics used to treat infection. This platelet clumping also causes small blood clots, growths on the heart valves, and inflammation of blood vessels that block the blood supply to the heart and brain. This further shows the connection between gum disease and heart disease, and how difficult it might be to treat it.

Because biofilms are highly resistant to antibiotics, and they are responsible for diseases such as ear infections, bacterial endocarditis (infection of the inner surface of the heart and its valves), cystic fibrosis, legionnaire's disease, and hospital-acquired infection from catheters, medical implants, wound dressings, and medical devices, it has become more important than ever to understand them. We strive to learn where they grow and how they affect us. From a dental perspective, it is important to know because biofilms are not only found in plaque, they can also grow on oral appliances such as dentures, mouth guards, and night guards, so it is important to follow all cleaning advice given by your dentist.

Clogged drains are also caused by biofilm, and you may have seen biofilm on slimy rocks when walking by a river. Biofilms also colonize household surfaces in the bath and kitchen. And, of course, the plaque that forms on your teeth and causes tooth decay and periodontal disease is a type of biofilm.

The build-up of plaque formed during the onset of gingivitis represents the overgrowth of bacteria as a biofilm on the teeth above and below the gum line. Biofilms can form in other parts of the body as well, and are known to be involved with health conditions such as urinary tract infections and chronic sinusitis. Researchers believe learning about how the body interacts with bacteria overgrowth during gingivitis could provide insight into a variety of biofilm-related diseases.

Oral biofilms are commonly associated with infections such as cavities, gingivitis, and periodontal disease. With antibiotic resistance continually on the rise, researchers are exploring alternative sterilization methods to effectively treat biofilms.

Blue light commonly used by dentists to cure resin fillings and hydrogen peroxide combined may be capable of reaching and treating bacteria in deep layers of biofilms that can cause cavities and gingivitis. Treatments like blue light and water ozonators are being investigated to purify the mouth before proceeding with traditional treatments such as scaling and root planing.

In a study on biofilms of Streptococcus, S. Mutans were exposed to wavelengths of visible light consisting of 400 to 500 nm for 30 to 60 seconds while in the presence of 3 to 300 mM of hydrogen peroxide. Microbial counts from each treated sample were compared with those of the control and results showed that visible light and hydrogen peroxide combined, successfully penetrated all layers of the biofilm, creating an antibacterial effect.

Removal of biofilm, better known as plaque, is important. Unfortunately some traditional methods of removal in the dentist office like vibration might be allowing the bacteria into the bloodstream, so we need pre-conditioning to reduce the population of bacteria before treatment.

The ozone generator purifier eliminates dental water biofilms. Just as plaque grows on the surface of teeth, bacterial biofilms grow on the walls of the tubing used to deliver water to the dental instruments, including the dental hand pieces used in cleaning and scaling. In order to not only clean the mouth, but also the instruments and tubing that delivers the water for treatment, I utilize oxygenated water treatment in my office. In fact, the oxygenated water is said to be more antibacterial than Chlorox...which to me is quite the claim!

Another product that we use in our office is Perio Protect. Perio Protect® is a new way to manage oral biofilm with minimal invasive procedures. It combines treatments such as chemical debriding therapy in conjunction with traditional mechanical procedures. The chemical therapy consists of a tray delivery of doctor-prescribed solutions to bring the medications directly to the periodontal pockets to disrupt the biofilm growth.

The normal procedures of scaling and root planing remove plaque and tartar and help reduce bacteria, but the bacterium then begins to reproduce and the biofilms regenerate, so it is difficult to control them between office visits. With Perio Protect® Method, the patient is given a customized dental tray and the solution to use between visits. In this way, we can help patients manage the growth of biofilm.

The most common solution also contains oxidizing and oxygenating agents, which are beneficial to good oral health. Many dentists are now choosing to treat with chemical solutions and cleansing agents before traditional debriding procedures to reduce bacterial populations because we understand the problems of introducing bacteria into the bloodstream now, and want to reduce the risk of that happening during mechanical debridement.

Another new treatment is the 10-64 wavelength laser specific to the red spectrum. Used in conjunction with oxygenated water treatment lasers could help reduce the biofilm structure before more invasive treatments are initiated.

Randy is a great example of the benefits of these new treatments. He had pockets that were too deep for him to maintain, and had potential for systemic disease. So we started with a procedure I call LARP, laser assisted root planing. It involves de-epethelialization of the pocket wall with the laser, followed by root planing and then irrigating with ozonated water. All of this is very comfortable and pain free. The result is less pocketing, and less risk for oral disease that can cause systemic disease.

Standard periodontal protocols

Unfortunately the dental industry has come under fire for an "unacceptable and growing chasm" between the care that's needed and what is actually being provided. As we learn more about the effects of poor oral health in the body's overall health, health care programs are changing to allow for better dental care, more often.

Many dentists today are talking about creating a standard of periodontal protocols. A system like this could help ensure that the misdiagnosis of periodontitis would become less common. As one article stated, "In today's dental climate, no hygiene department should be prophy based."

Creating a periodontal protocol with guidelines for annual probing and charting for all adult patients is an important first step toward delivering the current periodontal standard of care. This protocol could also instruct on further treatment required based on the probing and charting data. This would put all dentist offices on the same level of periodontal care, and ensure that the fight against gum disease was being met in a standard and effect way.

Periodontal protocols can be found online. Perhaps it is up to the individual to get educated! Knowledge is power, and knowing what effective periodontal protocol is, followed by the implementation of these treatments, could save your life.

Treatments for Gum Disease

The most obvious and basic first step of treatment for gum disease is the basic removal of biofilm, plaque, and calculus by way of scaling. This is performed by your dental hygienist or dentist. Once this is completed, follow-up care is important. Medications such as chlorhexidine gluconate, which comes in the form of a prescription mouthwash that helps kill the bacteria in your mouth, is the first line of defense in conjunction with good daily flossing and cleaning, and frequent checkups.

If the periodontitis has progressed, non-surgical and surgical options are both available to stop or minimize the progression of periodontal disease. Surgery can also be used to replace bone lost in the advanced stages of the disease.

Researchers have tested the efficacy of grape seed extract on the presence of biofilm. Dental plaque biofilm is impervious to antimicrobial agents, but they found the polyphenolic extract at a concentration of 2,000 ug/ml was successful in penetrating and depleting the biofilm.

Treatments and research are rapidly changing, but the most important point is to address the problem and be ready to embrace the new science behind the treatments.

Chapter Nine

Dentists/Physicians Unite

One day in the not-too-distant future the big picture of your state of health will be found in little pictures of the mouth. In fact, you may find yourself being tested for cardiovascular disease, plaque of the arteries, or even lung cancer in your dentist's chair.

The mouth is an excellent indicator of the whole body's health, and dentists are becoming more important to the overall health care community. Dentists are able to predict upcoming problems for patients based on what they see happening in the mouth.

The chair of the new Department of Oncology and Diagnostic Sciences at the University of Maryland Dental School, Li Mao, believes that pinpointing molecular changes in living tissue from the mouth is an important technology in cancer studies and biomarker discovery.

He says that 50% of oral cancer patients get diagnosed too late, and he feels that dental education and services need to be rethought to include more than just cleaning and filling teeth.

The Dean from the same university agrees with him. There needs to be a bridge between medicine and dentistry that hasn't existed before.

For example, future lung cancer trials could be designed so that surface tissues inside the cheek could be checked while you are at the dentist. This will enable us to diagnose mouth and lung cancer far sooner than normal practices allow.

So the next person who reminds you to floss might be your cardiologist instead of your dentist!

Dentists and Physicians Unite

A new paradigm between dentistry and medicine is now developing regarding patient care. As the oral systemic connection is more clearly understood, dentists who are trained in diagnosing oral and periodontal disease will play a greater role in the overall health of their patients. Many times, the first signs of unnatural systemic health conditions reveal themselves in changes within the oral cavity. Medical histories should be carefully reviewed when 'at risk' patients are identified. A comprehensive Periodontal Risk Evaluation should be performed and results should be sent to the patient's treating physician(s).

> *A new paradigm between dentistry and medicine is now developing regarding patient care.*

Physicians will play a more active role in the oral systemic connection. They will screen 'at risk' patients for the common signs of periodontal disease, which include bleeding gums, swollen gums, pus, shifting teeth, chronic bad breath, and family history of periodontal disease. When appropriate, they will refer them to Dentists and Periodontists who are uniquely qualified to evaluate and treat their patient's oral conditions. This new era of interdisciplinary dental/medical cooperation will undoubtedly result in improved patient health, as well as improvement in overall patient longevity.

Blood tests are now available to dentist offices to test you for high levels of C-reactive protein levels, diabetes risk, and cholesterol. Dentists are taking a new role in your medical health because they have the ability to predict these diseases through your oral care. It's happening now, where dentists and doctors are working more as a team.

A new screening diagnostic system called STAT-CK, developed by Dr. Neil R. Gottehrer, DDS, will give the dentist and the patient a simple solution to visualize and categorize the stages of periodontal disease using grades A through F (A being minor damage to gums, F being the most severe case of damage to the gums and bone, needing surgical attention). This diagnostic tool can be personalized for each patient, and it allows all doctors to understand the patient's periodontal condition. It will improve the communication between dentist and doctor and patient, a three-way communication where everyone will be on the same page regarding the patient's oral health.

Game changer: oral DNA labs

One of the new developments in the dental industry is the ability to perform specialty diagnostics through oral medicine. These clinical tests are performed by dentists by taking samples from your mouth. They are then sent to oral labs for testing, just as your blood test is sent to a lab for testing. This process, however, is showing promise for earlier detection of disease. This means catching things when they are easily treated!

The area of Salivary Diagnostics is one of the most exciting new frontiers of Healthcare. Soon your dentist will be able to do salivary diagnostics to assist in the diagnosis and treatment protocols for most systemic diseases. OralDNA˙ Labs is one of the first to pursue this mission. Using the most advanced laboratory diagnostics and a team of dedicated dental and laboratory professionals, OralDNA˙ Labs is a leader and pioneer in this field of oral diagnostics.

Chapter Ten

Refresh Your Mouth - Part 2

Proper Oral Care

After reading all of this, I think we can agree on the facts. Gum disease causes bad bacteria in the mouth, and gives it access to the rest of your body while triggering a chronic immune response that is unhealthy. The biofilm from that bad bacterium causes thickening of the arteries, which can lead to stroke

> "If you are not taking care of your mouth, then you are not taking care of your whole body and it will kill you." Whoopi Goldberg on ABC-TV's The View, Oct. 2008z

and heart disease. It reduces overall health, and may lead to other systemic diseases, costing you more money in health care. It can even affect your success at work and in relationships.

The great news is through proper oral care you can reverse the process of gum disease...with no symptoms! All it involves is removing tartar and cleaning plaque off the teeth. No surgery, no antibiotics, just basic cleaning and care of your teeth and gums. How simple is that?

However, if your gum disease has progressed enough that further treatment is required, it is important--life or death important--to seek that help. So let's talk more about solutions, proper care, and what it all looks like for you.

As we mentioned in chapter eight, scaling and root planing is the first treatment for periodontal disease. Scaling and root planing removes the biofilm and irritants under the gums to stop the process of inflammation and infection. During this procedure, the mouth is numbed so the hygienist can remove deposits and biofilm from below the gum line without causing you discomfort. This is the part called scaling, and it's like removing the scales from a fish. Most hygienists also use ultrasonic vibrating tools to help get these deposits off the teeth. This leaves a rough surface, so planing is needed.

> *ScienceDaily, March 4, 2007 - Scientists at University College London (UCL) have conducted the first clinical trial to demonstrate that an intensive treatment for periodontitis (gum disease) directly improves the health of blood vessels.*

Planing is just the same as what a woodworker does to smooth wood. The dental hygienist surgically planes the root surface. This allows the gums to regenerate without irritation. The gum tissue shrinks and tightens around the teeth because there is no longer anything irritating in the way. This also reduces bleeding gums.

After these processes, the gums heal. The results can be determined by charting the gum pocket depth, with a goal of 1-3mm depth.

Often this is the only treatment that is required. It is non-surgical, and highly effective for treating early periodontal disease because it eliminates the inflammation and infection that promotes the tissue destruction around the teeth. And, of course, relief of inflammation in the mouth through intensive treatment of periodontitis results in improved function of the arteries.

Weapons Against Disease

Now that the link between inflammation in the mouth and heart disease has emerged and been proven and accepted, we could see development of new treatments for the big killers (heart attack and stroke) and maybe even a drastic reduction in the numbers of people afflicted by these diseases. All we have to do is convince ordinary people to take care of their gums.

So your toothbrush becomes a weapon against heart disease. Remember, forgetting to brush twice a day raises your risk of heart disease by 70%, according to a study done with over 10,000 adults. Brushing more really matters. Scrubbing with fluoride toothpaste robs oral bacteria of sustenance. Frequent cleaning--ideally, right after every meal or snack--prevents buildup that can lead to gum disease. There are also great studies coming in on the effectiveness of the use of xylitol. I highly suggest looking into the website, www. zelliescleanwhiteteeth.com. It highlights "world changing" work in this area being done by Dr. Ellie Phillips. Be sure to use a soft-bristle brush, and be gentle to avoid hurting the gums.

Also note: proper tooth brushing involves spending more time than most people realize. It's important to brush for at least two minutes...that's 120 seconds! Take a timer into the bathroom and see if it seems an inordinately long time compared to what you usually do. Kids especially like this exercise, and are very surprised at how long two minutes feels while brushing.

Use short, gentle strokes. Pay attention to your gum line, not just the surfaces of the tooth itself. Be sure to get right in the back, in behind those last teeth in the row, and areas around fillings, crowns, or any other dental work.

And, yes, please replace your toothbrush at least every three months. Bacterium does build up. You might also want to replace your toothbrush after having a cold or flu, since the germs happily co-inhabit every little crack and crevice that the bacteria also like.

What about flossing, you ask? Well, if you forget to floss, you undermine all that work you just did while brushing. Only floss can reach below the gum line. Unchecked bacteria in the pocket between tooth and gum can cause inflammation, tissue damage, and bone loss. As we've discovered, that bacteria can then spread to the bloodstream and get carried to the rest of the body. Further, tooth loss is caused more often by gum disease than tooth decay. So for good looks and good health, you must brush *and* floss daily.

It may surprise you to discover that not all floss is created equal. Coated and tape floss are not as effective at catching onto the build-up as the yarn type of floss. If you use a floss holder or pre-strung dental floss, you must be sure the floss is held taut. Then, be sure to curve the floss around each side of the tooth and go right down beneath the gum line. Use a gentle back and forth motion to insert the floss and to remove it.

There are fantastic products that will assist you in both brushing and flossing. Motorized toothbrushes have improved the amount of plaque the regular user can remove by brushing alone. Hydro Floss® oral irrigator is a machine that uses a pulsating stream that flushes disrupted plaque that brushing and flossing have left behind.

A swish afterwards does help. Using an ADA-approved mouth rinse offers some decent benefits. Research shows that the antimicrobial rinses (and antimicrobial pastes) reduce bacterial count and will inhibit their activity. Fluoride rinses used along with fluoride paste give more protection against decay than fluoride paste alone.

If you are struggling with dry mouth problems due to prescription medications or other reasons, try Oxyfresh Mouthrinses. They contain Oxygene®, which dissolves odor-causing microorganism by attacking the sulfur compounds.

We need to oxygenate our mouths. There are oxygen loving bacteria and oxygen hating bacteria. Bad bugs do not like oxygen. Around healthy teeth we see a 1-3mm rubbery pocket along the side. Health bacteria--the kind we need for good health and digestion--live there and flourish with adequate oxygen reaching them. Then, as periodontal disease sets in, the pockets grow, and that reduces the oxygen. Now you have swelling, bleeding, and this affects the healthy bacteria while also providing a nice home for the nasty bacteria that causes disease throughout our bodies. At 6+mm there is a proven reduction in oxygen.

Be sure to also keep in mind your "pocket size" guide to periodontal health; periodontal pockets of one to three millimeters with no bleeding are not a concern but pockets of four millimeters and over may need a more in-depth cleaning called scaling and root planing.

All of these things are important to good care at home. Of course, you will still need some help along the way. Two or more yearly cleanings are crucial. Some plaque gets trapped below the gum line and hardens into tartar, irritating and inflaming the gums. Even good flossing won't make it budge; only your dentist can remove it.

There are new nutritionals available today to help with the process of improving oral health. Called nutriceuticals, these supplements contain grape seed extract. Pharmaden is the only one that underwent double blind testing to ensure product quality. According to their product information, it is "distilled in a very specific way so only low molecular weight esters (the best absorbed) are used."

As we discussed before, grape seed extract is a powerful anti-inflammatory and has antioxidant properties twenty times stronger than vitamin C. Most dentists advise those who just underwent scaling and root planing to take a supplement like this to help the immune system as the gums heal. There is also ground-breaking information being released on the positive effects of Vitamin D, Omega 3's, and various anti-oxidants such as Juice Plus and their reduction of gum disease and inflammation.

So, root planing and scaling will get things back on track. If you require this kind of treatment, be sure to follow up with good oral care at home and with regular checkups to ensure the bleeding and inflammation has stopped.

It is so exciting to me how simple the solution is. With this new approach and a refreshed life, we could see a significant improvement in our overall health, adding years to our life, and improving1` the state of our health care system.

Chapter Eleven

The Future: Old Model vs New Model

"The terms oral health and general health should not be interpreted as separate entities," says Donna I. Shalala, former Secretary of Health and Human Services. Oral health is integral to general health and is essential to the overall health and wellbeing of all individuals. The early identification of oral disease may contribute to the early diagnosis and treatment for a number of systemic diseases.

So we need to ask ourselves the question, "Why, When, Where, and How did the Mouth become separated from the rest of the body?"

History

First we must look back. In the early 1800's, almost all of the dental training came through trade-like apprenticeships. There were debates over whether dentistry should be taught as part of higher education or simply through trade schools. So in 1840, the first dental school offering the Doctor of Dental Surgery (DDS) degree was the Baltimore College of Dental Surgery, led by visionaries Hayden and Harris, bringing about the foundation for a formal education in the field of dentistry. A little over 20 years later in 1867, Harvard Dental School became the first university-based dental education, bringing the same academic status of higher education to dentistry. But at this time, the profession was still basing itself on a mechanical approach to the mouth.

In 1908, Vida A. Latham, both a dentist and physician, wrote about the need for medical education for dentists in dental schools. Latham was a health science pioneer, and one of the first to recognize the importance of medical education in dental education. Latham even went as far as suggesting that dentistry is a specialty of medicine. Latham also suggested that the practice of dentistry should be more scientific, and not merely mechanical. Even in 1908, she stated that unless the dental practitioner understood systemic disease and its inception, he or she could not accurately perform as a diagnostician.

Old Model

As the twentieth century progressed, we as a society often feared our dental visits, fighting trench mouth, pyorrhea (sounds like oral inflammation), loose teeth, gross decay, dentures, partials, bleeding gums, amalgam fillings, poor appearance, crooked teeth, and abscesses, to name a few. There was an understanding that if it did not hurt, there was nothing wrong. Nothing could be further from the truth! That was the "OLD MODEL".

But now we find Oral Health means more than the lack of pain. Oral Health means more than healthy teeth. The word "oral" refers to the mouth, including not only teeth and gums, but also the tongue, lips, salivary glands, hard palate, soft palate, mucosal lining of the mouth and throat, chewing muscles, and jaw.

New Model

Today we have the support of the mounting evidence showing the connection between our Oral Health and our General Health. So it's time for the "NEW MODEL".

New Model: Prevention

The "NEW MODEL" is a wellness model, no longer waiting for health to fail before it is addressed. The easiest path to health is to prevent disease, not repair disease.

Here are examples of what we now believe to be the criteria for a healthy mouth, thanks to my friends at NextLevel Practice;

- Pink Gums
- Gum pocket depths of 3mm or below
- No bleeding
- No cavities
- No decay
- No leaky fillings
- No fractured or chipped teeth
- No malocclusion or crowding
- No gum recession
- No sensitivity
- No oral cancer
- No crowded or missing teeth
- Fresh breath

From this baseline, we establish ORAL HEALTH.

New Model: Screening

The next step for the "NEW MODEL" involves the dentist and dental hygienists in the key role to screen patients for systemic disease and to provide the interaction and management with other areas of healthcare.

Salivary Diagnostics

One of the most exciting new areas of screening is through Salivary Diagnostics. There has been groundbreaking research in this area, revealing that saliva carries certain Biomarkers (signs) to reveal the potential for disease. Salivary Diagnostics quite often replaces invasive blood tests with a simple, non-invasive oral rinse. And recently, nanotechnologies have brought us advancements in screening and testing. Manufacturers and practitioners will eventually have access to portable devices to diagnose a variety of disease conditions, all easily obtained from an oral sample instead of traditional blood drawn tests. Much of the screening technologies that underlie these laboratory tests on saliva samples are based on Nobel Prize winning technology.

At first, many of the salivary diagnostics were directed at oral diseases. There are salivary tests for oral diseases such as dental decay, gum disease, and oral cancer. OralDNA labs has been a leader in this area. They have a simple salivary test for gum disease, a test for a person's genetic risk for gum disease, and a test for HPV and risk for oral cancers. The most exciting progress to date has been made in the area of oral cancer.

But now there are salivary diagnostics for Systemic Diseases. As we explore Systemic Disease, we have found many Disease Biomarkers (signs) that are transported through saliva from what is called "gingival crevicular fluid". There is a lot more taking place in terms of salivary diagnostics on the Systemic Disease front than on the Oral Disease side. There's work being done investigating markers (signs) for such Systemic Diseases as Cancer, Cardiovascular Disease, and Infectious Diseases. It's possible to measure C-Reactive Protein, known to reflect Arteriosclerosis and Heart Disease. We have oral tests for HIV, they are also working on TB and malaria. We are also seeing ground-breaking work on HPV, also known as human papillomavirus, which is associated with cervical cancer, and suspected to be involved in numerous other cancers.

In addition to salivary diagnostics, there are many other screening and diagnostic tools that are directly related to the affects of Oral Health on General Health. These include diabetic status and hemoglobin A1c testing, blood pressure, C-reactive protein levels, cholesterol testing, nutritional and antioxidant status, home studies for sleep apnea, TMJ/TMD screening, and safe heavy metals removal, to name a few.

Salivary diagnostics give dentists the ability to not only screen, but also diagnose diseases immediately. Dentists see patients more regularly than physicians, and therefore are in a unique position to screen for diseases and direct patients in the appropriate manner. It is not that the dental team would attempt any type of medical treatment. Rather it could ultimately expand the role of the dental team, not only in oral healthcare, but in expanding its role in improving everyone's general healthcare.

New Model: Communication

This NEW MODEL is also based on vastly improved communication between both dentist and patient, and dentist and MD.

It all starts with patient education. We can't fix what we don't understand. There is ground breaking work being done in this area. One of my favorite education tools is "My Health Report". My Health Report provides unique and important information, various resources, and educational videos that all help individuals lead healthier lives, reduce risk factors that lead to death and disease, and show individuals how to have a healthier mouth and smile. And the best part is "My Health Report" is customized for each individual. It starts with a simple group of health questions that assess an individual's health risks. From these health risk factors, a personalized health report is produced for the individual. It is provided online, with suggested resources for the individual to help themselves in the process. The outcome is a vastly improved individualized plan of care for each person. There are educational videos, short video clips indexed by topic to provide better understanding of various dental and medical related topics that affect your health. Also there are various articles, helpful links, and several additional resources. My Health Report also offers ground-breaking "health risk assessment calculators". These are a quick way to learn how health risk factors may be impacting your life. It helps you discover what's impacting your health and how reducing risk factors will keep you healthy.

The Communication with patients in the NEW MODEL is further improved with the advent of intraoral cameras, digital radiography, large computer monitors, and various audio visual enhancements.

The next key to communication in this NEW MODEL is vastly improved communication between Dentists and Physicians. It benefits all of us when Physicians are aware of the connection between gum disease and heart disease, diabetes, and cerebrovascular disease (stroke). It's also helpful for Physicians to be aware of the connection between migraines, facial pain and TMD. Further, it's helpful for Physicians to be aware that Dentists are treating patients using oral sleep appliances for the many people with sleep apnea that are CPAP intolerant. And most important is the Dentist understanding and being able to communicate with the Physicians.

In this NEW MODEL, Dentists will be called to a new and more collaborative role in healthcare. With the many new approaches to screening and diagnosing, there will be a need for a vastly improved system of communicating between the dental healthcare professionals and the various other healthcare professionals. There are currently systems that have been developed to utilize electronic communications directly between Dental and Medical Healthcare Professional. They are a secure, confidential, and safe way to carry out these all too important Communications.

New Model: The Experience

The final key to the NEW MODEL is the EXPERIENCE. The OLD MODEL EXPERIENCE was often one of pain, along with numerous assaults on the senses, and often based on a sickness model. The perception was if it didn't hurt, there was nothing wrong. Pain became the determining factor for treatment. And this became the basis for a whole society's view of Oral Health. Pain became ingrained in our public perception of Oral Health. Great progress has been made, but often the "perception" people have is of the 1950's version of dental care.

In the NEW MODEL, the EXPERIENCE is not just the reduction of pain, but creating an environment of comfort. No more assaults on the senses. First, we can change things by improving the sounds of the dentist office, replacing the old sounds of drills with soothing and healing surroundings, including the sound of flowing water. Next, the NEW MODEL is an open, airy environment with a light, bright, comforting feel. There is the elimination of the old tastes and smells, and the addition of pleasant new tastes and smells. The individual is also comforted with warm massaging chairs, soft blankets, and warm moist towels.

In the NEW MODEL, the individual has total control. The end result is an EXPERIENCE that is conducive to total health and wellness. It's a totally REFRESHING EXPERIENCE to REFRESH LIFE. The New MODEL is sustainable and GREEN!

New Model: The Purpose

The final piece of the NEW MODEL is the PURPOSE. The SOULFUL PURPOSE of the NEW MODEL is to help prevent heart attacks, stroke, diabetes, and other systemic diseases. These are diseases affected by inflammation. Everyone has an accumulation of these factors in their life that cause inflammation. The total of these factors is called "cumulative inflammatory burden". When the burden gets past a certain point that causes disease, it's called that person's "Tipping Point". By reducing oral disease and improving oral health, we help prevent inflammatory diseases such as heart attacks, stroke, diabetes, etc.

The end result of the NEW MODEL is to REFRESH LIFE!
The NEW MODEL is 'THE REFRESH LIFE CENTER'.

Chapter Twelve

Refresh Your Life

It is my hope that through what you know now you will change everything about the way you treat your mouth. Spread the word! Awareness and education will do so much to help people realize how important good oral care is to their very life. And further, not only can we prevent frightening diseases with good oral care, we can enjoy better overall whole body health. So refresh your life today, and tell the people you care about how they can too.

New solutions for better treatment are arriving every day, new innovations that will change the face of dental care and health care. We will see dentists and doctors working together to ensure you are getting the care you deserve. With awareness of our own role to play as well, we can all take the steps required to improve overall health worldwide!

The whole idea of the Refresh Life book is to open a door to your health, to show you the connections so that you understand how crucial it is to care for your teeth and gums. I truly feel this is the new 'no smoking' cry for health. Now that you know that bleeding gums can be a greater risk to your health than smoking, you can see why we need to get this message out there! Let people know that if they are not flossing and not caring for their oral health, it is the equivalent or worse than smoking a pack a day!

Today's dentists need to step up and take responsibility, too. We need to enforce zero tolerance for bleeding gums. We need to find ways to safely remove biofilm. We need to pay attention to all the research. We need new and innovative professional dental solutions. Most especially, we need to pay attention to this message!

Remember:

- Gum therapy improves blood vessel health and helps prevent heart attacks and stroke.
- Healthy Gums help prevent diabetes.
- Healthy Gums increase the chances of having a full term birth of healthy size.
- Healthy Gums have actually been shown to reduce wrinkles.
- Healthy Gums have been shown to reduce erectile dysfunction.

Dr. Oz states that regular flossing adds 6 1/2 years to your life. But it goes so much beyond that. We're talking years not spent in a hospital fighting disease. We're talking years of not being cared for by professionals because our mind is lost to Alzheimer's. We're talking extra years of good health to spend traveling or with your grandchildren or pursuing the dreams you put on hold as a younger adult.

We're also talking about lower health care costs worldwide, if we can get people to listen to this message. But all of it is dependent on each individual taking five minutes to floss, brush, and rinse, and unfortunately many people just don't. They don't understand how devastating the effects of gum disease can be on their very life.

Please remember the idea of 'mostly right most of the time.' Don't expect perfection as you take on new ideas and habits for better health. Make small changes, and work towards good flossing and brushing most of the time. If you forget or let it slide one night, don't let that be the reason you quit altogether. Mostly right most of the time. That's the way to make a difference over the long term.

So I urge you, the reader, the one now armed with knowledge and understanding, to go out and spread the word! We all deserve a good smile, and we all deserve great health.

Refresh your Life. Take the time for yourself with simple, easy, painless treatments to reverse whatever level of oral disease you currently have. It might just save your life.

The mouth is where life begins...let's not let it end there.

Refresh Life Bibliography of References

Toothbrushing Less Than Twice a Day Linked to Increased CV Risk
Heartwire CME, June 7, 2010
http://cme.medscape.com/viewarticle/723057?src=cmenews&uac=146410FN

Forget Botox. Floss your teeth.
By Lisa Zamosky
msnbc.com contributor msnbc.com contributor
updated 6/18/2010 8:25:41 AM ET
http://www.msnbc. msn.com/id/ 37692310/ ns/health- skin_and_beauty/

High Antibody Levels to *P.gingivalis* in Cardiovascular Disease
S. Bohnstedt, M.P. Cullinan, P.J. Ford, J.E. Palmer, S.J. Leishman, B. Westerman, R.I. Marshall, M.J. West, and G.J. Seymour
published 2 June 2010, 10.1177/0022034510370817

Stave Off Heart Disease? Brush Twice Daily.
By Megan Johnson
Posted: May 28, 2010http://health. usnews.com/ health-news/ family-health/ heart/articles/ 2010/05/28/ health-buzz- want-to- stave- off-heart- disease-brush- twice-daily. html

From Annals of Cardiac Anaesthesia (ACA):
Periodontal diseases: A risk factor to cardiovascular disease
Rajiv Saini[1], Santosh Saini[2], Sugandha R Saini[3]
[1] Department of Periodontology, Rural Dental College-Loni, Maharashtra, India
[2] Department of Microbiology, Rural Medical College-Loni, Maharashtra, India
[3] Department of Prosthodontics, Rural Dental College-Loni, Maharashtra, Indiahttp://www.annals. in/article. asp?issn= 0971-9784; year=2010; volume=13; issue=2;spage= 159;epage= 161;aulast= Saini

P. Gingivalis mechanism uncovered.
Source: University of Louisville
http://www.thefreelibrary.com/P.+Gingivalis+mechanism+uncover ed.%28health.%29-a0226218897

Healthy Mouth Standard; Next Level Practice

Scientists Find New Clues to Bacteria Responsible for Periodontal Disease
February 11th, 2010, By Dental Health Magazine Staff
http://worldental.org/dental-news/scientists-find-new-clues-to-bacteria-responsible-for-periodontal-disease/1088/

The Gums of Steel Intro Webinar
http://attendthisev ent.com/? eventid=11684451

Adding 6 Years to Your Life Through Flossing
By Patrice Barber
http://ezinearticles.com/?Adding-6-Years-to-Your-Life-Through-Flossing&id=3715846

Sharp Rise in HPV-Related Oropharyngeal Carcinoma -- A Legacy of the "Sexual Revolution"?
Medscape Medical News
http://mp.medscape.com/cgi-bin1/DM/y/eCxRF0XTfMI0F6E0K 55y0GV&uac=146410FN

Periodontal Bacteria Found In Amniotic Fluid
ScienceDaily (July 6, 2007)
http://www.sciencedaily.com/releases/2007/07/070703171912.htm

**Turn That Frown Upside Down: Healthy Gums Are
Something To Smile About**
ScienceDaily (Apr. 1, 2008)
http://www.sciencedaily.com/releases/2008/03/080331122538.htm

Healthy Smile May Promote a Healthy Heart
ScienceDaily (Jan. 9, 2008)
http://www.sciencedaily.com/releases/2008/01/080108114329.htm

Brush Your Teeth To Reduce The Risk Of Heart Disease
ScienceDaily (Sep. 11, 2008)
http://www.sciencedaily.com/releases/2008/09/080908203017.htm

**My Health Report; mydentaletc.com
Treatment For Gum Disease Could Also Help The Heart**
ScienceDaily (Mar. 4, 2007)
http://www.sciencedaily.com/releases/2007/03/070302111134.htm

**Shared Genetic Link Between Dental Disease Periodontitis
And Heart Attack Discovered**
ScienceDaily (May 25, 2009)
http://www.sciencedaily.com/releases/2009/05/090525105423.htm

**Periodontitis And Myocardial Infarction: A Shared Genetic
Predisposition**
ScienceDaily (Feb. 24, 2009)
http://www.sciencedaily.com/releases/2009/02/090213115011.htm

**History Of Periodontitis Linked To Cerebrovascular Disease
In Men**
ScienceDaily (July 3, 2009)
http://www.sciencedaily.com/releases/2009/06/090630163152.htm

Over Half Of People With Rheumatoid Arthritis Have Periodontitis
ScienceDaily (June 12, 2009)
http://www.sciencedaily.com/releases/2009/06/090612115429.htm

Patients With Moderate To Severe Periodontitis Need Evaluation For Heart Disease Risk
ScienceDaily (July 10, 2009)
http://www.sciencedaily.com/releases/2009/06/090630101332.htm

Link Between Oral Infections And Cardiovascular Disease Morbidity Explained
ScienceDaily (July 13, 2009)
http://www.sciencedaily.com/releases/2009/07/090709140822.htm

Inflamed Gums Linked To Heart Disease
ScienceDaily (Dec. 20, 2008)
http://www.sciencedaily.com/releases/2008/12/081215184308.htm

Blue Light And Hydrogen Peroxide May Effectively Treat Biofilms That Cause Cavities And Gum Disease
ScienceDaily (July 24, 2008)
http://www.sciencedaily.com/releases/2008/07/080722094227.htm

Nearly One Third of Human Genome Is Involved in Gingivitis, Study Shows
ScienceDaily (Dec. 9, 2009)
http://www.sciencedaily.com/releases/2009/12/091207123115.htm

Maintaining Healthy Teeth And Gums Is A Wise Investment
ScienceDaily (Feb. 5, 2009)
http://www.sciencedaily.com/releases/2009/02/090206094543.htm

Your Oral Health Is Connected To Your Overall Health
ScienceDaily (Apr. 11, 2009)
http://www.sciencedaily.com/releases/2009/04/090404093335.htm

Treating Gum Disease Linked To Lower Medical Costs For Patients With Diabetes
ScienceDaily (Jan. 8, 2009)
http://www.sciencedaily.com/releases/2008/12/081223172745.htm

Treating Your Periodontal Pockets May Benefit Your Pocket Book
ScienceDaily (Nov. 28, 2007)
http://www.sciencedaily.com/releases/2007/11/071127163734.htm

Mouth Is Indicator of Overall Health, Says Dental School Professor
ScienceDaily (Nov. 14, 2009)
http://www.sciencedaily.com/releases/2009/11/091113121410.htm

Effect of Periodontal Treatment on Glycemic Control of Diabetic Patients

1. Wijnand J. Teeuw, DDS[1],
2. Victor E.A. Gerdes, PHD[2,3] and
3. Bruno G. Loos, PHD[1]

http://care. diabetesjournals .org/content/ 33/7/e102. full

Medical Problems Caused by Rotten Teeth
By Susan Brassard
http://www.livestro ng.com/article/ 164883-medical- problems-caused-by- rotten-teeth/

The AAP Risk Assessment Test
http://service. previser. com/aap/default. aspx

3 Foods for Healthy Gums and Hearts
by Emily Sohn
http://www.kitchend aily.com/ 2010/06/24/ 3-foods-for- healthy-gums- and-hearts/

Toothbrushing Less Than Twice a Day Linked to Increased CV Risk
Heartwire CME , 2010-06-07
https://profreg.medscape.com/px/getlogin.do?urlCache=aH
R0cDovL2NtZS5tZWRzY2FwZS5jb20vdmlld2FydGljbGGU
vNzIzMDU3P3NyYz1lbWFpbHRoRoaXM=

Testing for HPV in the dentist's office
by KING 5 News
KING5.com - Posted on May 27, 2010 at 5:05 PM
http://www.king5. com/health/ Testing-for- HPV-in-the- dentists-
offices-95053669 .html

Adjunctive effects of a dietary supplement comprising dried whole fruit, vegetable and berry juice concentrates on clinical outcomes of treatment of periodontitis
Iain L. C. Chapple[1], Michael M. Milward[1], Nicola Ling-Mountford[1], Paul Weston[1], Gerard E. Dallal[2] and John B. Matthews[1]
[1] School of Dentistry, Periodontal Research Group, University of Birmingham, Birmingham, United Kingdom
[2] Biostatistics Unit, USDA HNRC at Tufts University, Boston, MA
http://www.fasebj.org/cgi/content/meeting_abstract/24/1_Meetin
gAbstracts/540.10?maxtoshow=&hits=10&RESULTFORMAT=&
fulltext=Chapple&searchid=1&FIRSTINDEX=0&volume=24&is
sue=1_MeetingAbstracts&resourcetype=HWCIT&eaf&eaf

The American Academy for Oral Systemic Health
http://www.aaosh.com/

Causal Link Between Periodontal Disease and Alzheimer's Disease?
Adapted from ScienceDaily for Perio Talk
http://www.perio-talk.com/2010/09/causal-link-periodontal-
disease-and.html

Key reason 'found' for gum and heart disease link
BBC News Health
http://www.bbc.co.uk/news/health-11182666

Dr. Oz Show Focuses on Patients with Sleep Disorders
Spotlight on 20 Million Americans with Sleep Apnea
January 21, 2010 11:28 AM Eastern Daylight Time
http://eon.businesswire.com/news/eon/20100121006172/en/ARES/
Dr.-Oz/John-Sculley

Cleveland Clinic Unveils "Top 10" Medical Innovations For 2010
CLEVELAND, Oct. 7, 2009
http://my.clevelandclinic.org/heart/news/archive/top_10_
innovations_2010.aspx?utm_campaign=emailfriend&utm_
medium=email&utm_source=ccf

Oral Health and Systemic Disease
California Dental Association
http://www.cda.org/popup/Oral_Health

Why "mouthless" medical schools?
N England Journal of Medicine.
Sognnaes RF. 1977;297(15):837-838.

The necessity of a medical education for dentists.
Dent Dig. 1908;14:425-426. Latham VA.

Primary health care assessment and intervention in the dental office.
Lamster IB, Wolf DL. J Periodontol. June 7, 2008.

Report of the independent panel of experts of The Scottsdale Project. Grand Rounds in Oral Systemic Medicine. Hein C, Cobb C, IacopinoA. 2007;2(3 Suppl):5-27.

9 781452 533575